Implantable Cardioverter-Defibrilator

Implantable Cardioverter-Defibrillator

A Practical Manual

by

L. Bing Liem

Stanford University Medical Center,
Stanford, CA, U.S.A.

KLUWER ACADEMIC PUBLISHERS
DORDRECHT / BOSTON / LONDON

A C.I.P. Catalogue record for this book is available from the Library of Congress.

ISBN 0-7923-6743-X

Published by Kluwer Academic Publishers,
P.O. Box 17, 3300 AA Dordrecht, The Netherlands.

Sold and distributed in North, Central and South America
by Kluwer Academic Publishers,
101 Philip Drive, Norwell, MA 02061, U.S.A.

In all other countries, sold and distributed
by Kluwer Academic Publishers,
P.O. Box 322, 3300 AH Dordrecht, The Netherlands.

Printed on acid-free paper

Printed in the Netherlands.

To Jim,

**whose patience and support
have made this writing possible**

Table of Contents

Foreword

At the dawn of the twenty-first century, ICDs have reached the mainstream of tachyarrhythmia therapy. Most ICD recipients have structural heart disease and receive ongoing care from cardiologists who are not electrophysiologists. Clinical cardiologists and heart failure specialists are increasingly involved in the prescription of ICD therapy and follow-up of ICD patients. If the indications for ICD therapy and the trend for ICD implantation without antecedent comprehensive electrophysiologic evaluation continue to increase – as seem likely – cardiologists may be increasingly involved in ICD implantation.

Comprehensive texts provide excellent references on ICD therapy for the expert electrophysiologist, but there remains a need for a succinct, focused, clinical text on ICD therapy both for the non-electrophysiologist and for fellows in cardiology or cardiac electrophysiology. Dr. Liem's Practical Manual fills this important role for cardiologists, fellows in cardiology, and physicians in other specialties who are required to treat ICD patients with increasing frequency, such as anesthesiologists, radiologists, intensivists, and emergency physicians. It could only have been written by a leading, experienced implanter and clear-thinking, hands-on clinician like Dr. Liem.

The Manual begins with succinct summaries of the place of ICDs in overall antiarrhythmic therapy and present clinical indications for ICDs. The section on Device Operation covers clinical application of basic physiologic and bioengineering principles relevant to defibrillation, basic cardiac pacing issues relevant to ICDs, as well as single-chamber and increasingly complex, dual-chamber tachyarrhythmia detection algorithms.

The Implantation Procedure section is a thorough guide for implanters, including details of ICD explantation and lead revision. The rapidly increasing simplicity of ICD implantation provides a stark contrast to the even more rapidly-increasing complexity of ICD programming and troubleshooting. Appropriately, the most comprehensive section of the Manual addresses patient management. The detailed, clear, and well-illustrated discussions of programming considerations and practical aspects of troubleshooting may prove to be the most valuable sections for clinicians involved in follow-up of ICD patients. Sections on drug and pacemaker interactions, electromagnetic interference, ICD radiography, and quality of life focus on how these subjects relate to clinical management.

This Manual provides a succinct guide to the basic principles guiding ICD therapy and a comprehensive approach to the management of ICD patients.

It should serve as an especially important resource for fellows in cardiology and non-electrophysiologists who participates in the care of ICD patients.

Charles D. Swerdlow, M.D.
Research Scientist II - Cedars Sinai Medical Center
Clinical Associate Professor of Medicine - University of California Los Angeles
Los Angeles, California

Introduction

Many significant developments in the field of medicine evolved from an intricate collaborative work between scientists, engineers, and clinicians. The progress of implantable cardioverter-defibrillator (ICD) therapy is of no exception. The idea was born from a clinician's desire to prevent sudden death and carried on to an early concept of a wearable and, eventually, potentially implantable defibrillator. The early struggles in conceptual and engineering feats were supported by dedicated scientists and clinicians and maintained by unrelenting preservation amidst some skepticism and criticism. The unyielding effort eventually resulted in the production of a solid device system with proven efficacy, practical applicability and comprehensive performance capability.

The developmental steps in the progress of ICD technology occurred as a result of an integrative effort between clinicians and engineers. The field was regarded as highly specialized and its application was expected to be limited only to the experts specializing in that field. However, as device implantation becomes progressively simpler and the application of therapy continues to evolve to include a much broader range of patients, it is inevitable that the general cardiologists become also closely involved in the selection and follow-up of the patients and, in some instances, the implantation procedure. Unfortunately, even though the application of the therapeutic concept has become simpler, the operation of the device has become more sophisticated and complex. The assumption that the clinical management of a patient with an ICD would be similar to that of a patient with a pacemaker would certainly be an erroneous and overly simplified one. The management of the patient with an ICD would, in the first place, pose a clinical challenge of understanding the operation of both a bradycardia and tachycardia device. The clinician should be familiar with the operation of these devices both as separate entities and as a unit. Additionally, the management of tachyarrhythmia prevention involves sudden death risk, and the consequences of any error are usually much less forgiving than of an inadequate programming of a pacemaker. Finally, the automation of tachyarrhythmia therapy does not always result in a simpler algorithm; in fact, the added features for tier-therapy and arrhythmia discrimination would pose the clinician with decision that would require a thorough understanding of the various arrhythmias.

The indication for ICD therapy is a continuing evolving concept. The scope of therapy for malignant ventricular tachyarrhythmia is an ever-changing one. The role of antiarrhythmic drug is constantly challenged. The concept of arrhythmia suppression was gradually replaced by a method utilizing cardiac electrophysiology (EP) study as well as empiric prescription of a "broad spectrum" antiarrhythmic drug such as amiodarone and sotalol. At the same time, data from clinical studies involving ICD indicate the superiority of device therapy and therefore, it is likely that secondary and primary prevention of arrhythmia will be managed primarily with an ICD. Even the role of EP study in the management of these patients is being challenged, both in terms of therapy selection and risk stratification. It is conceivable that the recommendation of ICD therapy is made on the basis of clinical criteria alone, without the involvement of the electrophysiologist. Thus, it is prudent that the clinicians from all disciplines to understand the clinical scope of ICD therapy and the complexity of its operation.

This publication is intended to expose those clinicians that are likely to be involved in the decision making for ICD therapy and its follow-up with a comprehensive knowledge of availability, capability and intricacy of such therapy. We believe that the historical view is of some importance, especially in placing the indication of such therapy in the proper perspective. The development of device and lead technology is also of great significance in the appreciation of the current units and the management of older models and will therefore be included also. Closely related to this topic is the implantation procedure, because it requires a thorough understanding and appreciation of the various units, leads and their general and unique operation. The choice of unit and system would obviously be based on the patient's need and the device's system scope of operation, and the clinician must make the clear decision and offer the options to the patient prior to the surgery. The most important portion of the book is, obviously, the clinical management of the patient with the device, and therefore, the bulk of the content is devoted to topics related to this subject. Finally, and not of least importance, are the non-medical issues, such as the technical, physical, psychological, social, economical, legal, and logistics factors of this "technological" therapy. The role of the patient and family as individuals is often only considered as an after thought and not given enough priorities. To include all of the psychological and social aspects of ICD therapy into the picture would undoubtedly require more than the clinicians involved in the care of the patient. The involvement of other health care providers, such as the arrhythmia nurse specialists and counselors, and technical specialists from the manufacturer, is not only of significant importance; it is mandatory. The economical impact, and burdens, of this form of therapy is not known yet, but the assumption of its significance has greatly influenced its application. The logistics of this therapy in the society is also being felt. All of these issues will be discussed to the extent of available scientific and anecdotal data.

At present, ICD technology has reached a level that is satisfactory to its purpose. It remains an effective therapy for the prevention of sudden death despite the addition of tiered therapy and arrhythmia discrimination features. It has also incorporated dual-chamber pacing with satisfactory performance, including rate-responsiveness and mode-switching. This stage of development is, in terms of general clinical application, optimal and has therefore set the new platform "basic" modern ICDs. This publication is intended to include all of the features incorporated in such a device. Variety exists among the different models and the general principle and key differences will be outlined. Future advancements of ICD technology will include, among many things, dual-chamber defibrillation treatment, pacing preventive therapy for atrial and ventricular arrhythmias, and electrical therapy for congestive heart failure. Further advancement in hemodynamic sensors will also likely be incorporated soon. Undoubtedly, further battery, capacitor, and lead technology will allow for smaller, more powerful, and longer lasting device. The basic concept and available technology on these subjects will also be discussed.

The aim of this publication is to review the practical aspects of this increasingly technical therapy, to examine the controversies of its application, and to discuss the dilemmas involved in its economic and logistic aspects. It is hoped that this review will enhance the clinician's awareness of and respect for the complexity of the device therapy, and will erase the stigmas involved in the recommendation of its application. In this era of rapidly progressing technology, it would be impossible to publish a review that will be complete and up to date in terms of the details in the most current and upcoming models. Every effort has been made to include specific information on the current technology and a general overview of upcoming features. However, confidentiality of ongoing research and clinical investigations precludes a more thorough discussion on certain subjects. Furthermore, this book is not intended to be a thorough review of the scientific, technical and engineering aspects of the concepts and operation of the device. Other publications are available for such purposes.

L. Bing Liem, D.O.
Director, Experimental Cardiac Electrophysiology
Stanford University Medical Center
Stanford, California

CHAPTER 1

HISTORICAL PERSPECTIVE

The Development of the Implantable Defibrillator

Initially, the idea of having an implanted device that would automatically deliver an electrical shock was considered unconventional, too extreme and undesirable. The concept was looked upon with some degree of disbelieve and its future was greatly doubted. In spite of such skepticism, the implantable defibrillator found a definite role in medicine, although its application was initially limited to those patients with recurrent cardiac arrest that are refractory to other forms of therapy. In such patients, the physician would have no choice because other forms of treatment have been exhausted. Undoubtedly, in following such algorithm, some patients would have died from their arrhythmia and never benefited from the device therapy. In that respect, sudden death from ventricular arrhythmia was common and, to some degree, an acceptable outcome.

The concept of an implantable defibrillator arose from, ironically, such a setting.[1] The inventor, Dr. Michel Mirowski, was struck by the death of his former chief, Dr. Harry Heller, from refractory ventricular tachyarrhythmia and subsequently he founded the idea of a rapid, effective therapy using an implantable device.[2-4] He slowly developed his idea at various institutions during his emigration from Poland to Israel and later to France, where the concept was first tested clinically. Dr. Mirowski finally came to the United States and worked together with a key investigator and personal friend, Dr. Morton Mower. The early prototype automatic defibrillator was designed and tested in the 1970s.[5] Although these early works showed promising results, many experts in the medical and engineering field were skeptical of the practicality of such a device for clinical use. Nevertheless, the concept was slowly gaining acceptance because the alternative would be a condition that is potentially lethal.[6-9]

A defibrillation system was then tested in humans, to patients undergoing coronary artery bypass grafting surgery at the Johns Hopkins University Hospital.[10] Interestingly, the first step of the experiment utilized an exclusively intracardiac system. Defibrillation was performed between a catheter at the right ventricular apex and another incorporated onto the bypass canulla in the superior vena cava. Successful defibrillation was accomplished with a low energy of 5-15 joules.[11] Although these experiments showed the potential of a transvenous model, the engineering of such a system was not quite feasible. There was a concern with the stability of such an electrode and its potential damage to the small area it delivers the defibrillation energy to. An alternative system that was noted to be very stable and reliable was one using insulated patch electrodes

placed directly on the heart.   It took several years and many steps of
corroborative work with a manufacturer, Medrad Inc. (which later became Intec
Systems) of Pittsburgh, Pennsylvania, before an implantable prototype was ready
and tested in dogs. The report included the classic motion picture showing the
rapid sequence of induction and conversion of ventricular fibrillation, with the
dog fully recovered and ambulatory within a few minutes.[12]

The first human implantation of the first complete automatic defibrillator
prototype was also performed at the Johns Hopkins University Hospital on
February 4, 1980.[13] The patient is a young woman who was referred by Dr.
Roger Winkle (who was then at Stanford University), and the team included,
among others, Dr. Phil Reed, Dr. Morton Mower, and Dr. Levi Watkins. These
prototype units and second-generation models incorporating cardioversion
therapy for ventricular tachycardia were implanted in the clinical investigation
phase, which ran through 1982, at the Johns Hopkins University and Stanford
University Hospitals.

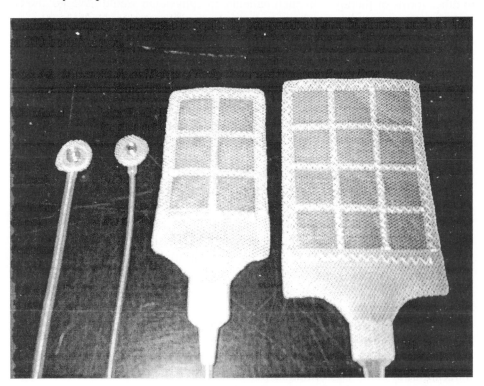

Figure 1-1. Shown here are the typical epicardial leads used in the early days of ICD implantation.
The system consisted of epicardial patches (small or large, right) and two epicardial screw-in leads
(left).

These early generation ICD models were implanted using epicardial
patches and screw-in leads (Figure 1-1), which became the standard lead system
for many years to follow. Such a system was chosen based on prior trials using

others, including an endocardial system. As defibrillation and lead/electrode technology was still limited in those years, the best approach was believed to be one which involve sandwiching the heart, including the left ventricle, with a large-surface electrode. The standard operation involved a thoracotomy (usually via left lateral thoracotomy approach), which in it self carried a modest risk and therefore patient selection was partly influenced by surgical risk stratification. Candidates for ICD, at that time, were those with recurrent cardiac arrest in whom choices of antiarrhythmic drugs had been exhausted. Hence it would not be surprising that the data from the first 52 patients was striking (Figure 1-2), showing a significant reduction of sudden death and total mortality.[14] Obviously, such an uncontrolled study and others[15-18] that used historical data or symptomatic firing as surrogates for mortality received criticism, but nonetheless the results were still considered promising.

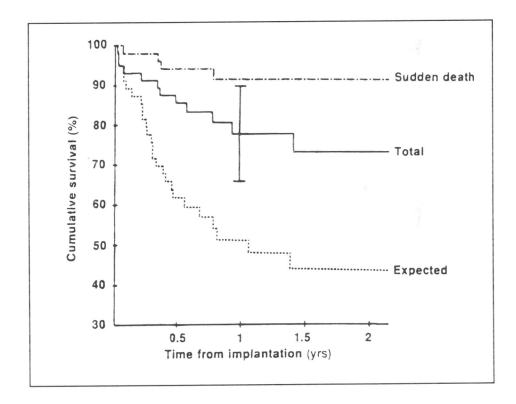

Figure 1-2. The survival curves in the first 52 patients. Sudden death and total mortality curves are actual survival curves while the expected curve was derived from symptomatic firings of the devices (reproduced with permission from Singer I, (ed) Implantable cardioverter-Defibrillator. Armonk, NY: Futura Publishing Company, Inc; 1994).

The device received approval from the Food and Drug Administration (FDA) in 1985 and was subsequently marketed by Cardiac Pacemakers

Incorporated (CPI) and its parent company, Eli Lily and Company, which acquired Intec System in 1985. The device was given the trade name of Automatic Implantable Cardioverter-Defibrillator (AICD). The survival data from the AICD patients also showed a significant reduction in arrhythmic death. Furthermore the data showed an improvement in the survival of patients with the device compared to those in the earlier study using AID. This difference was thought to be due to the more responsive AICD units, both in terms or recognizing arrhythmia (VT instead of VF) and response time (e.g., typically 17 seconds instead of 36 seconds).

> **Even early experience using the first ICD model showed the efficacy benefit of this therapy modality in reducing sudden death mortality. The survival benefit was maintained and slightly improved with subsequent models**

Other manufacturers also introduced implantable devices in the late 1980s; and this era marked the exponential growth of new implantation. The general term Implantable Cardioverter Defibrillator (ICD) was introduced to incorporate devices other than the AICD.

> - The concept and initial design of implantable defibrillator was initiated by Dr. Michel Mirowski and was first clinically implemented at Johns Hopkins University Hospital in 1980.
> - First clinical result of implantable defibrillator therapy was published in 1983, showing it's potential benefits in reducing recurrent sudden death and overall mortality.
> - The AICD received FDA approval in 1985.

Other Therapy for Ventricular Tachyarrhythmia

The progress in ICD clinical utility occurred in the wake of increasing appreciation of the magnitude of sudden death syndromes. Efforts for controlling ventricular tachyarrhythmia were also evident through the developments of newer antiarrhythmic drug and surgical therapies. Even in the present era of wide spread use of ICD, alternative therapy is at time necessary, and the role of such therapy has to be placed in its appropriate perspective.

Drug Therapy

Drug therapy played in important role in the management of patients with ventricular tachyarrhythmia. In spite of current data favoring the use of ICD, drug therapy remains a viable alternative and can be used in many circumstances. Furthermore, antiarrhythmic drug can be very useful as an adjunct therapy for reducing ICD shock therapy and for the management of atrial arrhythmias. A large portion of patients that underwent ICD implantation is also given antiarrhythmic drugs for those reasons.

Drug Therapy as the Sole Treatment for Ventricular Tachyarrhythmia

The method for selecting the appropriate drug for the treatment of VT/VF has been a topic of debate in the past two decades and controversies remain with regard to the best approach. Perhaps the only clear conclusion is the recommendation against empiric use of (Vaughan-Williams) Class I (sodium-channel blockers) antiarrhythmic drugs.[19-21] Empiric use of some other drugs such as amiodarone and sotalol, however, may be reasonable. For sodium-channel blockers, the selection of their use should be more individualized, using an index of arrhythmia presence in the drug-free state and then assess the ability of a drug to suppress it. This can be done non-invasively using ambulatory monitoring or invasively using intracardiac electrophysiology study.

> Antiarrhythmic drugs remain useful for the management of VT/VF but their utility and method of selection should be individualized

The Non-Invasive Method

The method for selecting antiarrhythmic drug therapy using the noninvasive approach was popularized by Lown and coworkers.[22] A drug-free study using ambulatory monitoring is used for baseline, which must show frequent spontaneous ventricular arrhythmia, in the form of single premature ventricular complexes (PVCs, 30 per hour for at least 50% of the time) and nonsustained runs of > 3 beats. Alternatively, an exercise stress test can be used if it reproducibly induce VT or VF. The definition for satisfactory suppression on drug therapy is not standardized but in general, investigators agree that it should include at least 50% suppression of PVCs, 90% suppression of couplets, and complete elimination of nonsustained runs of > 3 beats.

Several studies have evaluated the outcome of patients with therapy predicted to be effective by this approach to those with therapy predicted ineffective or received empiric treatment.[23] In general, the studies showed that the noninvasive method is able to stratify the outcomes. The patients treated with drugs selected by this method generally have a favorable two-year sudden death recurrence of 8-18%, compared to 40% in the other group. Using this method, approximately 40% would not qualify because of lack of spontaneous ventricular arrhythmia on ambulatory monitoring or lack of VT/VF inducibility on exercise treadmill test. Nevertheless, the data support the utility of this method in selecting antiarrhythmic drug treatment.

The Utility of Electrophysiology Study and Programmed Stimulation

The field of cardiac electrophysiology has provided the clinician further insight into the mechanism of cardiac arrhythmia and tools for better management and therapy assessment. In the field of ventricular tachyarrhythmia, programmed electrical stimulation (PES) method was considered particularly useful because it is an effective and accurate method for assessing reentry VT[24-

[31], the most common form of VT in patients with an underlying chronic ischemic heart disease and a prior scar from myocardial infarction.

The PES method, which uses rapid ventricular pacing followed by up to three extrastimuli at progressively shorter coupling intervals, induces reentrant VT by encountering relative refractoriness, slow conduction and unidirectional block.[24,32-34] In utilizing this method, one should be aware of its limitations. One limitation is the fact that triggered activity, a type of tachycardia that resulted from afterdepolarizations, can also be induced using rapid pacing. However, several features of a triggered activity rhythm can be used to distinguish it from a reentry one. In general, a triggered activity form of tachycardia can also be readily initiated with fixed cycle length pacing which is less likely to induce a reentry form. When a triggered activity form is initiated using extrastimulus method, there is usually a direct or parallel relationship between the coupling interval of the extrastimulus to the interval between the extrastimulus and the first tachycardia impulse. In contrast, an inverse relationship is usually present in the initiation of a reentry rhythm. Furthermore, the extrastimulus method rarely initiates a sustained triggered activity rhythm. It is important to be certain that the arrhythmia initiated at the EP study is not a triggered activity VT because ICD is not an appropriate therapy for this form of arrhythmia. Such form of VT usually self terminates and rarely requires cardioversion therapy. Moreover, triggered activity VT may be cathecolamine sensitive and would likely to be aggravated by the occurrence of an ICD shock.

> **EPS is useful not only for the confirmation of diagnosis but to also rule out other VT mechanism which may preclude the use of ICD**

Another limitation in the PES method is related to its sensitivity and specificity. The likelihood of initiating a reentry rhythm increases with the use of more extrastimuli and shorter coupling interval. However, the use of an "aggressive" method with more than three extrastimuli and with very short coupling intervals reduces it specificity.[35-43] The optimal method is with the use of up to three extrastimuli and with coupling intervals of no less than 180 milliseconds. Yet another limitation is the possibility that the stimulus from the pacing catheter may not reach the reentry site, either due to too much conduction block in the intervening tissue or at the site of stimulation.[32] Such a case can be overcome with high intensity pacing, but this method can also initiate arrhythmia with questionable clinical significance.[44] It is recommended that pacing be performed at current twice diastolic threshold but not exceeding to 5 mA and up to 2 ms pulse width. If VT could not be induced from the usual right ventricular apical and outflow tract positions, pacing from the left ventricle should be considered. These considerations should be entered into the algorithm in recommending an ICD therapy. Thus, for example, the induction of VF in a patient with syncope and minimal structural heart disease would not be a strong indication for an ICD. In contrast, the failure to induce VT in a patient who has had documented VT should not hinder the decision for recommending ICD therapy.

Finally, the morphology of the induced arrhythmia may play a role in the interpretation of the study. An inducibility a monomorphic VT which can be reset, entrained or terminated with pacing indicates the presence of a "stable" reentry substrate. On the other hand, the induction of polymorphic VT or ventricular fibrillation (VF) is considered less specific, because such an arrhythmia can be induced even in a person without structural heart disease or a history of VT/VF.[38,43,45] Further difficulties are encountered in the interpretation of such situation where the clinical, presenting arrhythmia is also polymorphic VT. It would be difficult to determine whether the induced arrhythmia represents the clinical arrhythmia. In fact, such doubt can also be cast in the case of the induction of monomorphic VT, because frequently its morphology is different from the presenting VT.[34,38] It is also noteworthy that in most cases, the presenting arrhythmia is not documented in the form of a 12-lead ECG recording. Thus, overall, the issue of reproducing the clinical arrhythmia remains evasive. One should include such uncertainty in the decision of therapy recommendation.

Clinical Studies Using PES Method

Even with its notable deficiencies, PES has been shown repeatedly to be a useful method for the selection of antiarrhythmic drugs, especially in patients with an underlying chronic ischemic heart disease. Shortly after it was noted that PES was a useful method in inducing reentry arrhythmia reproducibly, several groups of investigators applied the technique for selecting drug therapy for patients with VT, VF or cardiac arrest. Several preliminary studies were published in late 1970s and other investigators published the results of their larger series in early 1980s.[46-49] In a landmark study involving over 200 patients, Swerdlow et al[48], reported that the patients who received EP-guided drug treatment had a sudden death rate of 18% at two years, compared to 41% in those who were treated by other methods. In this study, as is the case with many other similar ones, the independent predictive factors were the patient's NYHA status and persistent inducibility of VT/VF.

Even without the use of randomized method or a placebo control arm, those studies were well accepted and used as guidelines for the application of this method in clinical practice. The strength of these studies lies in the consistency of their results. The outcome of the patients treated with EP-guided method was always better than that of the patients treated by other methods. Also, the control group would typically have an outcome similar to that of historical control, as described by Liberthson et al, and Cobb et al, with a sudden death recurrence rate of approximately 25-30% after one year and 40-45% at two years.[6,50] Most importantly, multivariate analysis of clinical variables in these studied typically identified PES as an independent predictor of outcome.

Thus, the standard method of the management of chronic ischemic patients with a cardiac arrest or sustained VT episode was to identify potential efficacious drug therapy using PES method. For patients with a non-ischemic cardiomyopathy, the data were not uniform and the role of PES was marginal at best. In one of the few studies involving such a group of patients, it was shown that in those patients with reproducibly inducible VT, PES was also a useful method[49]. However, only less than 20% of patients entered into the study could benefit because in the remainder of patients, VT was either not induced or not reproducibly induced, or no drug was found to be effective.

> **EP-guided drug therapy for VT/VF is more appropriate than empiric use; however, the subset of patients that were found to be drug responders is typically small, < 50% in CAD patients and < 20% in IDCM patients.**

Non-Invasive versus Invasive Methods

The relative usefulness of the noninvasive and invasive methods were assessed in the ESVEM study (Electrophysiology Study Versus Electrocardiographic Monitoring Trial).[51-54] The 486 patients, most with chronic ischemic disease, were randomized and assigned to serial drug testing using ambulatory monitoring or EP study. The drugs used were imipramine, mexiletine, procainamide, quinidine, sotalol, pirmenol, and propafenone. Efficacy was predicted in 45% of the EP-tested versus 77% non-invasively tested patients and was predicted quicker in the non-invasive group. To the dismay of invasive method proponents, there was no significant difference in outcome in the two groups with the exception of lower arrhythmia recurrence at one year. Among the drugs used, sotalol had the lowest actuarial probability of arrhythmia recurrence, cardiac death, and overall mortality. The one surprising outcome is the high arrhythmia recurrence rate in both groups, which was speculated to be due to non-uniform method of PES.

Empiric Amiodarone Therapy

For the patients who are "non-responders", the treatment was usually empiric. In such a case, amiodarone is the most commonly used drug, because its presumed better safety and efficacy profile over other drugs. Amiodarone is also the ideal choice for an empiric therapy because, given its complex pharmacokinetics, an EP assessment would not be practical. The data from several early studies utilizing empiric amiodarone therapy are encouraging, showing a relatively low two-year sudden death mean rate of 12%.[55-58] In the CASCADE (Cardiac Arrest in Seattle: Conventional versus Amiodarone Drug Evaluation) study, empiric amiodarone therapy was tested against EP- and ambulatory monitoring-guided drug therapy in 228 survivors of out-of-hospital cardiac arrest.[59,60] At two years, there was a slightly lower mortality in the amiodarone group.

Amidst the vast need for an alternative drug treatment for patients who could not be suppressed by an antiarrhythmic drug using either the non-invasive or invasive method of selection, amiodarone found an important role. Later, the efficacy of empiric amiodarone was also tested against ICD therapy. In all of the studies (see below), ICD was found to be superior but in one study, CIDS (Canadian Implantable Defibrillator Study), the difference did not reach statistical significance.

> **Empiric amiodarone may be the best alternative to ICD therapy, even compared to EP-guided drug selection**

Antiarrhythmic Drug as Adjunct Therapy

Antiarrhythmic drug can be very useful as adjunct therapy. Patients with ICD often experience multiple therapies and those who have frequent shocks can be severely affected psychologically. In addition, a significant portion of patients with ICD also have atrial tachyarrhythmias that may need to be suppressed with antiarrhythmic drugs. Thus, in such patients, antiarrhythmic drug is usually prescribed. For such a purpose, a broad range of drugs could be used. The choice would typically depended on the status of underlying cardiovascular status and the drug's adverse effect profile. Thus, drugs with low proarrhythmic and negative inotropic effects (such as mexiletine) would frequently be selected. However, a relatively weak antiarrhythmic drug may not be adequate for suppression of atrial fibrillation or flutter. Alternatively, drugs with low side effect profile, such as propafenone, may be preferred. Sotalol and other class III agents, on the other hand, offer other advantages such as DFT lowering effect[61,62] and therefore, they might be the best drugs as an adjunct therapy in patients with ICD. In a randomized study involving 302 patients with ICD, sotalol was found to lower the incidence of death of any cause and delivery of first shock.[63] Beta blocker alone has been shown to be effective at reducing the incidence of arrhythmia in ICD patients. In a study comparing metoprolol to sotalol, metoprolol was noted to be more effective than sotalol in reducing the incidence of ventricular arrhythmia and in improving overall survival.[64] In that regard, amiodarone, even with its known potential deleterious effect on DFT, is also commonly used.

> **Antiarrhythmic drugs can be very useful for reducing arrhythmia frequency in ICD patients and some drugs, such as beta blockers, may further improve overall survival**

Therapy with antiarrhythmic drug will likely continue to play an important role in the management of patients with sustained VT/VF although it will mostly be as adjunct therapy.

- Antiarrhythmic drug therapy was a predominant mode of treatment in the management of patients with VT/VF.
- Drug therapy can still be useful for VT/VF but if used as a sole modality, its efficacy should be monitored, either non-invasively (by Holter or ETT) or invasively (with EPS) except for amiodarone
- EPS was found to be useful in identifying responders to drug therapy but it can be applied mostly to patients with underlying ischemic heart disease. In patients with underlying idiopathic cardiomyopathy, EPS failed to induce or reproduce sustained VT.
- EPS is still useful in identifying VT that may not be appropriate for ICD therapy (such as automatic/triggered-activity VT) and those that may be curable with catheter ablative therapy (such as automatic/triggered-activity VT, idiopathic VT, or BB-reentry VT).
- The ESVEM trial showed little differences in the outcome between patients managed with noninvasive method versus those managed with invasively. It showed that among the drugs used (imipramine, mexiletine, procainamide, quinidine, sotalol, and pirmenol), sotalol yielded the lowest actuarial recurrence of arrhythmia and mortality.
- The CASCADE trial showed empiric amiodarone therapy had slightly lower mortality compared to EP-guided and Holter-guided drug therapy.

Surgical Therapy

Surgical therapy for VT/VF also played a significant role in the progress of the disease management and in the appreciation of the disease process. However, data from surgical procedures are far fewer than its medical counterpart because the procedure could only be performed in select patients and was only available in a few medical centers.[65-70]

A specific, curative surgical therapy for ventricular tachyarrhythmia is performed with the aim of eliminating the "site" of reentry. In general, this is achieved by eliminating the scar (endocardial resection) and its borders. Indeed, reentry usually originates at the zone of incomplete infarction, where there exist areas of slow conduction and therefore, removal of ventricular aneurysm or the scar alone would not be beneficial. To assist the surgeon in identifying the site(s) of reentry, a pre-operative mapping is useful. This can be done by identifying a general focus based on the VT morphology on ECG or by endocardial mapping during an induced VT in the EP laboratory. However, as could be expected, in many instances, there were more than one "origin" identified during mapping.

Hence, a comprehensive VT surgery would include aneurysmectomy, endocardial scar resection, and cryoablation of some border zone sites. Cryoablation is also advantageous for areas where resection can not be performed, such as the papillary muscles or sites near the mitral valve annulus. As an alternative, an encircling procedure (encircling endocardial ventriculotomy) can be performed. The choice of the type of procedure performed usually depends on the center's experience.

The biggest draw back of surgical therapy is its morbidity and associated mortality. The relatively long procedure requires for mapping and meticulous resection and cryoablation pose a high morbidity risk. Furthermore, the extensive surgical removal of ventricular tissue may cause a significant burden to the left ventricle in the early recovery period, especially if no concomitant revascularization is performed. In this respect, a mechanical advantage would only be achieved in patients with a significant amount of dyskinetic aneurysmal wall segments. Thus, surgical therapy for VT is most beneficial for patients with distinct aneurysm and those who do not require a significant amount of mapping. It is perhaps for this reason also that the outcome in patients with posterior and inferior aneurysms, which would be more difficult technically to remove without jeopardizing the papillary muscles, was worse than that in patients with anterior wall aneurysm. It has been reported that carefully selected patients can be successfully treated with such a "blind" aneurysmectomy.[71,72]

The result of VT surgery has been variable, probably owing to differences in the method used, respective center experience, and patient population. The cumulative data from the Surgical Ablation Registry was reported in 1987. The Registry involved 8 centers from five countries with a total of 665 patients. Overall surgical mortality was 12% with 7 patients (1.1%) died intra-operatively. The overall post hospital discharge arrhythmic event recurrence was 16%. Antiarrhythmic drugs were used in 35.3% of patients surviving the surgery. Long-term overall survival was 72% after two years and 57% after five years (Figure 1-3). The underlying degree of cardiac dysfunction, as could be expected, was found to be a strong predictor of survival. Those patients (n = 50) with an LVEF of 40% or greater had a low (less than 5%) perioperative mortality and a five-year survival of greater than 90% while those with lower LVEF had high early and late mortality rates with a survival of < 60% after five years.

Post-operative electrophysiology study was useful in identifying patients who were still at risk for VT/VF. In the subgroup of 56 patients in whom the "clinical" VT was induced post-operatively, there was 41% recurrence rate of sudden death. The subgroup of 30 patients in whom "non-clinical" VT was induced had as good as an outcome (13% recurrence) as the 244 patients in whom no VT was inducible at all (12% recurrence). In many studies, patients with persistent inducibility of any VT would later undergo ICD implantation. In this respect, the VT surgery provided a preparation for the epicardial ICD system.

Conversely, because the surgical risk for thoracotomy-based ICD alone is also not trivial, VT surgery is frequently contemplated.

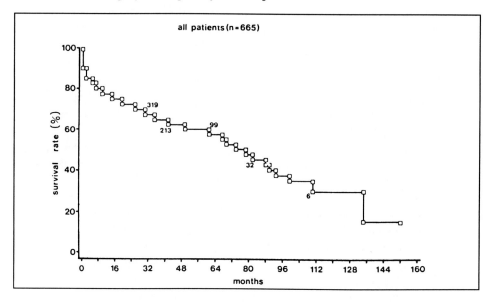

Figure 1-3. Overall survival of patients who underwent surgery for VT. Data were accumulated from the centers involved in the Surgical Ablation Registry (Reprinted with permission from Borggrefe et al.[73]

On the other hand, with its curative potential, VT surgery was, at one time, regarded as the preferred procedure. In the Stanford experience[69], over 100 patients underwent EP-guided VT surgery with a good overall outcome. The highest surgical mortality occurred in elderly patients and in patients with advanced heart failure. With the exclusion of those patient groups, the surgical mortality was approximately 5% and the success rate was 85%. Of those benefiting from long-term cure, the improvement in overall quality of life was excellent. In general, patients were able to return to or even gain better quality of life and employability. This aspect of the outcome may be significant from the patient's point of view and is frequently overlooked.

In the present era of simplified ICD implantation procedure, VT surgery is, in general, no longer the preferred choice. Even in centers that continue to perform this procedure, patients are carefully screened and only those with a distinct aneurysm and have the need for concomitant revascularization are considered. In limiting the candidates to these qualifications, arrhythmia surgery may indeed remain encouraging and will likely serve as a viable alternative to ICD therapy.

> **Arrhythmia surgery for VT is effective but carried a high morbidity and mortality rate; however, if performed in carefully selected patients, its benefits may be greater than those from ICD**

For most patients and in most instances, VT surgery is now considered as too risky. Furthermore, it is well recognized that in most patients suffering from VT, there are usually more than one site or region of "origin" and hence, even with accurate mapping, elimination of the "most likely origin of VT" would still leave the patient with potential other sites. ICD therapy would still be needed for such a scenario. However, if a patient were to undergo aneurysmectomy for indications other than VT, it would be beneficial for that patient to have the site of "clinical" VT mapped and removed. In such a scenario, whereby the remainder of the left ventricle is usually well preserved, VT may indeed be curable. With such careful screening and patient selection, VT surgery may carry low morbidity and mortality risks and the results can be quite rewarding. In centers outside the U.S., where ICD therapy is considered costly, such arrhythmia surgery may have a significant role.

- Curative surgery for VT is performed by aneurysmectomy, endocardial resection of scar and cryoablation of border zones and areas that could not be resected. It can be performed with or without EP-mapping.
- VT surgery can be associated with significant operative morbidity and mortality. It is probably most beneficial for patients with discrete anterior wall aneurysm.
- Many patients still require ICD implantation post-operatively because of persistent inducibility of VT.

The Emerging Role of the Implantable Defibrillator

In the realization of the limitations of therapy with antiarrhythmic drug and the relatively high risk of antiarrhythmic surgery, the implantable defibrillators started to gain a greater role in the management of patients surviving sudden death or sustained VT. Although the device was far from versatile at that early stage and its implantation was at times associated with significant morbidity, therapy implantable defibrillator was considered as the most reliable in terms of preventing recurrent sudden death.

The thoracotomy approach was the standard surgical procedure (Figure 1-4) (see also Chapter 4). As such, the procedure was associated with typical chest and pulmonary morbidity and the patient would normally be monitored in the Surgical Intensive Care units. Thus, the overall hospitalization of such a patient was quite prolonged because prior to undergoing the surgery, the patient would typically have gone through several antiarrhythmic drug testing. The hospitalization might also be prolonged by a waiting time if the device must first be "custom-ordered" from the manufacturer. Nevertheless, an increasing number of patients were implanted with the device because of its proven efficacy.

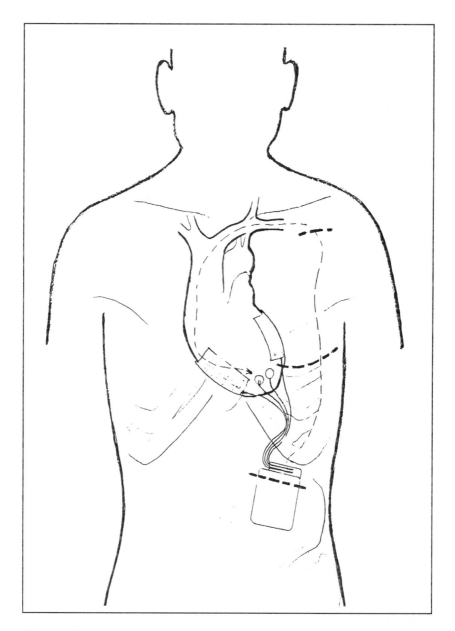

Figure 1-4. A diagram of a typical ICD system performed using thoracotomy approach. The epicardial patches and leads system are implanted directly onto the heart and then tunneled through the diaphragm to the abdominal area. The ICD generator is then implanted either subcutaneously or submuscularly in the left upper quadrant. If the pace/sense leads could not be implanted epicardially, a transvenous electrode (interrupted thin line) can be used and tunneled subcutaneously. The surgery requires at least a thoracotomy and an abdominal incision (interrupted thick lines).

As it was increasingly recognized that antiarrhythmic drugs were of limited value in this patient population, implantation of ICD became more "stream-lined" and, coupled with improved surgical experienced, the therapy became more acceptable. Thus, even though its role remained "last resort" and the surgery remained slightly risky for many years thereafter, ICD therapy became an important component in the algorithm of the management of patients with sustained ventricular tachyarrhythmias.

Subsequent AICD progress involved the development of a transvenous lead with a long defibrillation coil and a fixation mechanism similar to a transvenous pacemaker lead. With its significant technological progress, ICD has overcome many of its shortcomings and as a consequence, became the preferable form of therapy for ventricular tachyarrhythmias.

The modern ICD is equipped with tier-therapy, various bradycardia pacing modes and, recently, therapy for both atrial and ventricular tachyarrhythmias. In fact, the ongoing improvement and changes in its function has made it difficult to assign specific "codes" to the function of the device. At present, the following nomenclature is used by the North American Society of Pacing and Electrophysiology (NASPE) and British Pacing and Electrophysiology Group (BPEG)[74]:

I	II	III	IV
Shock Chamber	ATP Chamber	Detection Mode	Pacing Chamber
0 = none	0 = none	E = electrogram	0 = none
A= atrium	A = atrium	H = hemodynamic	A = atrium
V = ventricle	V = ventricle		V = ventricle
D = dual (A+V)	D = dual (A+V)		D = dual (A+V)

The simple nomenclature was created in 1993 and was derived from the one used for pacemaker. Interestingly, detection using hemodynamic mode was considered even at such early stage. Such mode may indeed be useful and some progress has been made in it (see also Chapter 6). At the present time, the typical, "complete" dual-chamber ICD would be labeled VVED.

References

1.   Mirowski D. Personal comments written about Michel Mirowski on behalf of the family. Pacing Clin Electrophysiol, 1991;**14**(5 Pt 2):872.

2.   Mirowski M, Mower MM, Staewen WS, et al. Standby automatic defibrillator. An approach to prevention of sudden coronary death. Arch Intern Med, 1970;**126**(1):158-161.

3.   Mirowski M, Mower MM, and Mendeloff AI. Implanted standby defibrillators. Circulation, 1973;**47**(5):1135-1136.

4.   Mirowski M, Mower MM, Gott VL, et al. Feasibility and effectiveness of low-energy catheter defibrillation in man. Circulation, 1973;**47**(1):79-85.

5.   Mirowski M, Mower MM, Staewen WS, et al. Automatic defibrillation. Jama, 1971;**217**(7):964.

6.   Cobb LA, Baum RS, Alvarez Hd, *et al.* Resuscitation from out-of-hospital ventricular fibrillation: 4 years follow-up. Circulation, 1975;**52**(6 Suppl):III223-235.

7.   Schaffer WA and Cobb LA. Recurrent ventricular fibrillation and modes of death in survivors of out-of-hospital ventricular fibrillation. N Engl J Med, 1975;**293**(6):259-262.

8.   Graboys TB, Lown B, Podrid PJ, *et al.* Long-term survival of patients with malignant ventricular arrhythmia treated with antiarrhythmic drugs. Am J Cardiol, 1982;**50**(3):437-443.

9.   Gillum RF. Sudden coronary death in the United States: 1980-1985. Circulation, 1989;**79**(4):756-765.

10.   Langer A, Heilman MS, Mower MM, *et al.* Considerations in the development of the automatic implantable defibrillator. Med Instrum, 1976;**10**(3):163-167.

11.   Mirowski M and Mower MM. Transvenous automatic defibrillator as an approach to prevention of sudden death from ventricular fibrillation. Heart Lung, 1973;**2**(6):867-869.

12.   Mirowski M, Mower MM, Langer A, *et al.* A chronically implanted system for automatic defibrillation in active conscious dogs. Experimental model for treatment of sudden death from ventricular fibrillation. Circulation, 1978;**58**(1):90-94.

13.   Stack JM, Houston C, Mirowski M, *et al.* Automatic implantable defibrillator for the patient with recurrent refractory malignant ventricular arrhythmias: case report. Heart Lung, 1982;**11**(6):512-515.

14.   Mirowski M, Reid PR, Winkle RA, *et al.* Mortality in patients with implanted automatic defibrillators. Ann Intern Med, 1983;**98**(5 Pt 1):585-588.

15.   Mirowski M, Reid PR, Mower MM, *et al.* Clinical performance of the implantable cardioverter-defibrillator. Pacing Clin Electrophysiol, 1984;**7**(6 Pt 2):1345-1350.

16.   Winkle RA, Mead RH, Ruder MA, *et al.* Long-term outcome with the automatic implantable cardioverter- defibrillator. J Am Coll Cardiol, 1989;**13**(6):1353-1361.

17.   Fogoros RN, Elson JJ, Bonnet CA, *et al.* Efficacy of the automatic implantable cardioverter-defibrillator in prolonging survival in patients with severe underlying cardiac disease. J Am Coll Cardiol, 1990;**16**(2):381-386.

18.   Cohen TJ, Reid PR, Mower MM, *et al.* The automatic implantable cardioverter-defibrillator. Long-term clinical experience and outcome at a hospital without an open-heart surgery program. Arch Intern Med, 1992;**152**(1):65-69.

19.   Vaughan Williams EM. Quantitative assessment of antidysrhythmic drugs. G Ital Cardiol, 1972;**2**(1):157.

20.   Vaughan Williams EM. Subgroups of class 1 antiarrhythmic drugs. Eur Heart J, 1984;**5**(2):96-98.

21.   Vaughan Williams EM. Significance of classifying antiarrhythmic actions since the cardiac arrhythmia suppression trial [see comments]. J Clin Pharmacol, 1991;**31**(2):123-135.

22.   Lown B. Management of patients at high risk of sudden death. Am Heart J, 1982;**103**(4 Pt 2):689-697.

23.   Lown B, Podrid PJ, De Silva RA, *et al.* Sudden cardiac death--management of the patient at risk. Curr Probl Cardiol, 1980;**4**(12):1-62.

24.   Josephson ME, Horowitz LN, Farshidi A, *et al.* Recurrent sustained ventricular tachycardia. 1. Mechanisms. Circulation, 1978;**57**(3):431-440.

25.   Horowitz LN, Josephson ME, Farshidi A, *et al.* Recurrent sustained ventricular tachycardia 3. Role of the electrophysiologic study in selection of antiarrhythmic regimens. Circulation, 1978;**58**(6):986-997.

26.   Horowitz LN, Vetter VL, Harken AH, *et al.* Electrophysiologic characteristics of sustained ventricular tachycardia occurring after repair of tetralogy of fallot. Am J Cardiol, 1980;**46**(3):446-452.

27.   Denes P, Wu D, Dhingra RC, *et al.* Electrophysiological studies in patients with chronic recurrent ventricular tachycardia. Circulation, 1976;**54**(2):229-236.

28.   Fontaine G, Guiraudon G, Frank R, *et al.* Modern concepts of ventricular tachycardia. The value of electrocardiological investigations and delayed potentials in ventricular tachycardia of ischemic and nonischemic etiology (31 operated cases). Eur J Cardiol, 1978;**8**(4-5):565-580.

29.   Josephson ME and Horowitz LN. Electrophysiologic approach to therapy of recurrent sustained ventricular tachycardia. Am J Cardiol, 1979;**43**(3):631-642.

30.   Josephson ME, Kastor JA, and Horowitz LN. Electrophysiologic management of recurrent ventricular tachycardia in acute and chronic ischemic heart disease. Cardiovasc Clin, 1980;**11**(1):35-55.

31.   Garan H and Ruskin JN. Localized reentry. Mechanism of induced sustained ventricular tachycardia in canine model of recent myocardial infarction. J Clin Invest, 1984;**74**(2):377-392.

32.   Gillis AM, Winkle RA, and Echt DS. Role of extrastimulus prematurity and intraventricular conduction time in inducing ventricular tachycardia or ventricular fibrillation secondary to coronary artery disease. Am J Cardiol, 1987;**60**(7):590-595.

33. Hammill SC, Sugrue DD, Gersh BJ, *et al*. Clinical intracardiac electrophysiologic testing: technique, diagnostic indications, and therapeutic uses. Mayo Clin Proc, 1986;**61**(6):478-503.

34. Josephson ME, Horowitz LN, Farshidi A, *et al*. Recurrent sustained ventricular tachycardia. 4. Pleomorphism. Circulation, 1979;**59**(3):459-468.

35. Spielman SR, Farshidi A, Horowitz LN, *et al*. Ventricular fibrillation during programmed ventricular stimulation: incidence and clinical implications. Am J Cardiol, 1978;**42**(6):913-918.

36. Morady F, Hess D, and Scheinman MM. Electrophysiologic drug testing in patients with malignant ventricular arrhythmias: importance of stimulation at more than one ventricular site. Am J Cardiol, 1982;**50**(5):1055-1060.

37. Stevenson WG, Wiener I, and Weiss JN. Comparison of bipolar and unipolar programmed electrical stimulation for the initiation of ventricular arrhythmias: significance of anodal excitation during bipolar stimulation. Circulation, 1986;**73**(4):693-700.

38. Stevenson WG, Weiss J, and Oye RK. Selecting therapy for sustained ventricular tachycardias: importance of the sensitivity and specificity of programmed electrical stimulation for predicting arrhythmia recurrences. Am Heart J, 1990;**119**(4):871-877.

39. Michelson EL, Spielman SR, Greenspan AM, *et al*. Electrophysiologic study of the left ventricle: indications and safety. Chest, 1979;**75**(5):592-596.

40. Farshidi A, Michelson EL, Greenspan AM, *et al*. Repetitive responses to ventricular extrastimuli: incidence, mechanism, and significance. Am Heart J, 1980;**100**(1):59-68.

41. Vandepol CJ, Farshidi A, Spielman SR, *et al*. Incidence and clinical significance of induced ventricular tachycardia. Am J Cardiol, 1980;**45**(4):725-731.

42. Cooper MJ, Hunt LJ, Palmer KJ, *et al*. Quantitation of day to day variability in mode of induction of ventricular tachyarrhythmias by programmed stimulation. J Am Coll Cardiol, 1988;**11**(1):101-108.

43. Hummel JD, Strickberger SA, Daoud E, *et al*. Results and efficiency of programmed ventricular stimulation with four extrastimuli compared with one, two, and three extrastimuli. Circulation, 1994;**90**(6):2827-2832.

44. Morady F, Dicarlo LA, Jr., Liem LB, *et al*. Effects of high stimulation current on the induction of ventricular tachycardia. Am J Cardiol, 1985;**56**(1):73-78.

45. Cua M and Veltri EP. A comparison of ventricular arrhythmias induced with programmed stimulation versus alternating current. Pacing Clin Electrophysiol, 1993;**16**(3 Pt 1):382-386.

46. Breithardt G, Seipel L, Abendroth RR, *et al*. Serial electrophysiological testing of antiarrhythmic drug efficacy in patients with recurrent ventricular tachycardia. Eur Heart J, 1980;**1**(1):11-24.

47. Morady F, Scheinman MM, Hess DS, *et al*. Electrophysiologic testing in the management of survivors of out-of-hospital cardiac arrest. Am J Cardiol, 1983;**51**(1):85-89.

48. Swerdlow CD, Winkle RA, and Mason JW. Determinants of survival in patients with ventricular tachyarrhythmias. N Engl J Med, 1983;**308**(24):1436-1442.

49. Liem LB and Swerdlow CD. Value of electropharmacologic testing in idiopathic dilated cardiomyopathy and sustained ventricular tachyarrhythmias. Am J Cardiol, 1988;**62**(9):611-616.

50. Liberthson RR, Nagel EL, Hirschman JC, *et al*. Pathophysiologic observations in prehospital ventricular fibrillation and sudden cardiac death. Circulation, 1974;**49**(5):790-798.

51. The ESVEM trial. Electrophysiologic Study Versus Electrocardiographic Monitoring for selection of antiarrhythmic therapy of ventricular tachyarrhythmias. The ESVEM Investigators. Circulation, 1989;**79**(6):1354-1360.

52. Biblo LA, Carlson MD, and Waldo AL. Insights into the Electrophysiology Study Versus Electrocardiographic Monitoring Trial: its programmed stimulation protocol may introduce bias when assessing long-term antiarrhythmic drug therapy. J Am Coll Cardiol, 1995;**25**(7):1601-1604.

53. Mason JW, Marcus FI, Bigger JT, *et al*. A summary and assessment of the findings and conclusions of the ESVEM trial. Prog Cardiovasc Dis, 1996;**38**(5):347-358.

54. Reiter MJ. The ESVEM trial: impact on treatment of ventricular tachyarrhythmias. Electrophysiologic Study Versus Electrocardiographic Monitoring. Pacing Clin Electrophysiol, 1997;**20**(2 Pt 2):468-477.

55. Fogoros RN, Fiedler SB, and Elson JJ. Empiric amiodarone versus "ineffective" drug therapy in patients with refractory ventricular tachyarrhythmias. Pacing Clin Electrophysiol, 1988;**11**(7):1009-1017.

56. Di Pede F, Raviele A, Gasparini G, *et al*. [Empiric treatment with amiodarone in patients with sustained ventricular tachyarrhythmia. Results of a long-term follow-up]. G Ital Cardiol, 1990;**20**(9):819-827.

57. Nora M and Zipes DP. Empiric use of amiodarone and sotalol. Am J Cardiol, 1993;**72**(16):62F-69F.

58. Proclemer A, Facchin D, Vanuzzo D, *et al*. Risk stratification and prognosis of patients treated with amiodarone for malignant ventricular tachyarrhythmias after myocardial infarction. Cardiovasc Drugs Ther, 1993;**7**(4):683-689.

59.   Randomized antiarrhythmic drug therapy in survivors of cardiac arrest (the CASCADE Study). The
       CASCADE Investigators. Am J Cardiol, 1993;**72**(3):280-287.
60.   Greene HL. The CASCADE Study: randomized antiarrhythmic drug therapy in survivors of cardiac
       arrest in Seattle. CASCADE Investigators. Am J Cardiol, 1993;**72**(16):70F-74F.
61.   Dorian P, Newman D, Harris L, *et al.* Sotalol in patients with implanted automatic defibrillators:
       effects on defibrillation and comparison with amiodarone. Can J Cardiol, 1994;**10**(2):193-200.
62.   Dorian P, Newman D, Sheahan R, *et al.* d-Sotalol decreases defibrillation energy requirements in
       humans: a novel indication for drug therapy. J Cardiovasc Electrophysiol, 1996;**7**(10):952-961.
63.   Pacifico A, Hohnloser SH, Williams JH, *et al.* Prevention of implantable-defibrillator shocks by
       treatment with sotalol. d,l-Sotalol Implantable Cardioverter-Defibrillator Study Group [see
       comments]. N Engl J Med, 1999;**340**(24):1855-1862.
64.   Seidl K, Hauer B, Schwick NG, *et al.* Comparison of metoprolol and sotalol in preventing
       ventricular tachyarrhythmias after the implantation of a cardioverter/defibrillator. Am J Cardiol,
       1998;**82**(6):744-748.
65.   Ostermeyer J, Breithardt G, Kolvenbach R, *et al.* Intraoperative electrophysiologic mapping during
       cardiac surgery. Thorac Cardiovasc Surg, 1979;**27**(4):260-270.
66.   Guiraudon G, Fontaine G, Frank R, *et al.* [Encircling endocardial ventriculotomy in the treatment of
       recurrent ventricular tachycardia after myocardial infarction]. Arch Mal Coeur Vaiss,
       1982;**75**(9):1013-1021.
67.   Breithardt G, Seipel L, Ostermeyer J, *et al.* Effects of antiarrhythmic surgery on late ventricular
       potentials recorded by precordial signal averaging in patients with ventricular tachycardia. Am Heart
       J, 1982;**104**(5 Pt 1):996-1003.
68.   Klein H, Frank G, Werner PC, *et al.* [Results of electrophysiologically guided surgery in ventricular
       tachycardia]. G Ital Cardiol, 1983;**13**(4):318-322.
69.   Swerdlow CD, Mason JW, Stinson EB, *et al.* Results of operations for ventricular tachycardia in 105
       patients. J Thorac Cardiovasc Surg, 1986;**92**(1):105-113.
70.   Saksena S, Hussain SM, Gielchinsky I, *et al.* Intraoperative mapping-guided argon laser ablation of
       malignant ventricular tachycardia. Am J Cardiol, 1987;**59**(1):78-83.
71.   Nath S, Haines DE, Kron IL, *et al.* The long-term outcome of visually directed subendocardial
       resection in patients without inducible or mappable ventricular tachycardia at the time of surgery. J
       Cardiovasc Electrophysiol, 1994;**5**(5):399-407.
72.   Thakur RK, Guiraudon GM, Klein GJ, *et al.* Intraoperative mapping is not necessary for VT surgery.
       Pacing Clin Electrophysiol, 1994;**17**(11 Pt 2):2156-2162.
73.   Borggrefe M, Podczeck A, Ostermeyer J, *et al.*, *Long-term results of electrophysiologically guided
       antitachycardia surgery in ventricular tachyarrhythmias: A collaborative report on 665 patients*, in
       Nonpharmacological Therapy of Tachyarrhythmias, G. Breithardt, M. Borgreffe, and D. Zipes,
       Editors. 1987, Futura Publishing Company: Mount Kisco, NY. p. 109-132.
74.   Bernstein AD, Camm AJ, Fisher JD, *et al.* North American Society of Pacing and Electrophysiology
       policy statement. The NASPE/BPEG defibrillator code. Pacing Clin Electrophysiol,
       1993;**16**(9):1776-1780.

CHAPTER 2

INDICATIONS FOR ICD THERAPY

Early Role of ICD

The role of ICD therapy has broadened significantly since its first clinical use in the early 1980s[1]. In its early era, ICD therapy was considered last resort and reserved only for patients with recurrent VT/VF that was refractory to drug therapy or arrhythmia surgery. It was not uncommon that patients would suffer recurrent cardiac arrest episodes before being considered for an ICD therapy. Such reluctance in prescribing an ICD therapy stemmed from several factors. The one foremost factor was that the concept was new, lacking clinical data and considered unusual and also somewhat undesirable. To have a rescuing form of therapy was considered unacceptable and inferior to drug or surgical therapy. Other factors were merely logistical ones. The device was not readily available and its implantation required an open chest operation, either a thoracotomy or sternotomy. Such an operation carries a small but not insignificant morbidity and mortality rate, especially in the typical VT/VF patients and thus further limiting the application of ICD therapy.

However, it was also becoming evident that there was no effective form of therapy for the prevention of sudden death. Drug therapy guided by electrophysiologic study was found to be applicable to only less than half of VT/VF patients with underlying ischemic heart disease[2-4] and a small fraction of those with idiopathic dilated cardiomyopathy.[5] Surgery for VT by the method of ventricular aneurysmectomy with or without adjunctive cryosurgery was suitable only for patients with discrete scar and good residual left ventricular contractility, and even in this selected group of patients, arrhythmia surgery was only successful in two thirds of the recipients.[6-10] In the wake of such realization, ICD therapy began to gain a broader acceptance as an alternative form of therapy for VT and VF, and its clinical application further expanded as it became increasingly available and simpler to implant. Within a few years, ICD therapy transformed from a treatment of last resort to the treatment modality of choice for the management of malignant ventricular tachyarrhythmia.[11]

Results of Clinical Trials

Early clinical studies using retrospective data showed that ICD patients had a very low sudden death rate of 2% a year with a cumulative rate of less than 10% at 5 years; far better than any protection from antiarrhythmic drug or surgery.[12,13] However, these studies contained some limitations. The result of these studies were considered to have overestimated device benefits because the study design frequently used the incidence of device therapy episodes, which might have included treatment for non-fatal arrhythmia as surrogate mortality events. But subsequent studies which included devices with memory features for the identification VF or rapid VT, confirmed the excellent success of conversion of such arrhythmia at greater than 98% rate, and further showed a significant projected survival benefit compared to the untreated populations.[14-16] Later, similar studies showed the benefit from ICD therapy was superior to that of empiric amiodarone or EP-guided drug treatment.[17,18]

Recently, several randomized studies were completed (Table 2-1). These studies specifically addressed the value of ICD therapy as compared to antiarrhythmic drug in a controlled, randomized fashion.[19-27]

Table 2-1. Recent trials involving ICD therapy and their results in terms of ICD benefit

Trial	Patients	Therapy	ICD Benefit
Secondary Prevention Trials			
AVID 1997	Syncopal sustained VT or VF and EF<40% (N = 1016)	ICD vs drug (empiric amiodarone or EP-guided sotalol)	↓ mortality with ICD at 18 months (p<0.02) (15.8±3.2% vs 24.0±3.7%)
CIDS 1998	VT/VF/syncope with induced VT (N = 659)	ICD vs amiodarone	↓ mortality trend with ICD at 3-yr (by 19.6%, p=NS) [22% crossed over to ICD]
CASH 1998	SustainedVT/VF (N = 346)	ICD vs drug (empiric amiodarone, propafenone or metoprolol)	↓ mortality with ICD (12.1% vs 19.6%, p=0.047) [propafenone arm closed after 1-yr due to ↑ death]
Primary Prevention Trials			
MADIT 1996	Post-MI with NSVT (3-30 beats), EF<35%, induced sustained VT off & on procainamide (N = 196)	ICD vs conventional (80% with amiodarone)	↓ mortality in ICD group (54% reduction, p = 0.009)
CABG-Patch 1997	CABG patients with EF<35%, (+) SAECG (N = 1055)	ICD vs control	No mortality benefit from ICD
MUSTT 1999	CAD, NSVT, EF<40%, induced sustained VT (N = 704)	EP-guided drug/ICD vs standard	↓ mortality with EP-guided ICD (12% vs 18% at 24 mos 25% vs 32% at 60 mos)

Secondary Prevention Trials

Results of large multi-center randomized secondary prevention trials, which used the broader and more definitive end-point of total mortality further underscored the importance of ICD therapy in these high-risk patients. Two of three major trials showed similar results. The AVID (Antiarrhythmics Versus Implantable Defibrillator) trial, considered as the landmark US trial, compared ICD to drug therapy (either empiric amiodarone or sotalol) in patients with clinically documented hypotensive VT and VF.[20,28] It showed a 39% reduction (p<0.02) in mortality with ICD compared with drug treatment after one year, 27% after two years, and 31% after three years. A counterpart study conducted in Germany, CASH (Cardiac Arrest Study Hamburg), which, like AVID, enrolled only VT/VF survivors, showed a 37% reduction (p=0.047) in mortality with ICD compared to empiric amiodarone or metoprolol.[21,25] Of note, in this study, the drug therapy arm initially also included propafenone but this treatment arm was terminated early due to excessive mortality. In a similar but not comparable third trial, CIDS (Canadian Implantable Defibrillator Study), which included a broader scope of patients such as those with syncope, there was only a modest 19.5% reduction (p=NS) in total mortality with ICD compared to drug (empiric amiodarone) after 3 years.[23,24]

The AVID study compared 507 patients who received an ICD to 509 patients who received either empiric amiodarone or EP/Holter-guided sotalol. The CASH study involved smaller number of patients in each arm and perhaps therefore showed only marginal benefit of ICD. At the time of its interim publication in 1998, the analysis included 56 patients who received propafenone, 56 amiodarone, 50 metoprolol, and 59 ICD. Its enrollment has exceeded 300 patients since. All drugs in the study were prescribed empirically. Total mortality was 12.1% in the ICD arm and 19.6% in the drug group (excluding propafenone, which was discontinued because of excess mortality compared with ICD). The CIDS trial included 659 patients who were randomized to either ICD or empiric amiodarone therapy. The study population in the CIDS trial was different from those in AVID and CASH in that it included patients with syncope and inducible VT.

The strength of these studies is not only reflected in their statistical power. These studies have significant clinical relevance because they involve the typical patients referred for possible ICD implantation and the drug therapy, such as a beta blocker, sotalol or amiodarone are the ones that would be normally considered as alternative. Also, the ICDs used in these studies were mainly implanted trough the transvenous approach (95% in AVID ICD arm).

> **The results of recent large randomized trials, AVID, CASH and CIDS, which showed that ICD was better than drug therapy in lowering mortality in VT/VF patients confirmed prior smaller studies**

Another secondary prevention trial, known as the "Dutch Study"[18], also compared the outcome between ICD (n= 29) and drug (n =31) therapies in patients who had a cardiac arrest and had inducible sustained VT or VF at four to 12 weeks after myocardial infarction. This study differs from the other studies in that there were smaller number of patients involved and that there were more antiarrhythmic drugs tested. After a median of 729 days of follow up, there were four deaths in the ICD arm and 11 in the drug arm. The difference did not meet statistical significance (p = 0.07) but still showed the relative advantage of ICD over drug. The strength of this study is the cost saving noted in the ICD arm.

Primary Prevention Trials

Attention was also given to primary prevention of sudden death from VT/VF. It is evident that in spite of increasing availability and responsiveness of mobile medical care, a large proportion of patients suffering from out-of-hospital cardiac arrest still died in the field. Based on available data, it is estimated that less than one third of these victims are successfully resuscitated by bystanders and paramedics and of those who are admitted to a medical facility, another large proportion died during their hospitalization. The fact that in many patients, cardiac arrest is due to VT/VF underscores the importance of primary prevention. Several key trials addressing the role of ICD therapy for the management of high-risk patients have recently been completed.

In the CABG Patch trial, where patients undergoing coronary artery bypass grafting (CABG) with a left ventricular ejection fraction LVEF of < 35% and positive signal-averaged electrocardiogram (SAECG) also received ICD patches and randomized to ICD or no therapy, there was no observed benefit from therapy. However ICD therapy was shown to reduce mortality in two other large trials.[22,29-32] The MADIT (Multicenter Automatic Defibrillator Implantation Trial) showed that in post myocardial infarction (MI) patients who had LVEF of < 35%, nonsustained VT, and inducible sustained VT not suppressible with procainamide, ICD therapy reduced mortality by 54% compared with conventional therapy.[19,33-35] In MUSTT (Multicenter UnSustained Tachycardia Trial), where post-MI patients with LVEF < 39%, nonsustained VT and inducible sustained VT were randomized to either no therapy or therapy with either ICD or EP-guided drug, it was shown that ICD therapy was better than either no therapy or EP-guided drug therapy.[26,27]

The MADIT study was also a landmark study in primary prevention of sudden death and was the first multicenter randomized trial to be completed. The study analyzed 95 patients in the ICD arm and 101 patients in the drug arm with total mortality as the end point. The result of the study showed a remarkable 54% survival benefit of ICD. However, there were some criticisms to the study. Drug therapy, although consisted largely of amiodarone, also included a variety of other antiarrhythmic drugs with known proarrhythmic potentials, which might have contributed to the higher mortality in this arm. The other main concern with the study is that beta blocker use was more prevalent in the ICD arm than in the drug arm and might have therefore contributed to the lower mortality rate in this group. Hence, even with its remarkable results, the MADIT study was viewed with some degree of skepticism. However, these concerns gradually resolved as the results of other trials were released.

> **Data from primary prevention studies, which also showed that ICD was a better therapy for lowering mortality in patients at risk for VT/VF further confirmed the usefulness of the therapy and provide us with a more effective modality for early sudden death prevention**

Thus, even though there were some differences in the outcome from the trials, the overall results suggest that ICD therapy is the most efficacious in terms of sudden death prevention and mortality reduction. The relatively modest benefit from ICD therapy in CIDS is thought to be due to inclusion of a lower risk group of patients with syncope but without documented VT/VF. Similarly, the lack of benefit from ICD in the CABG Patch trial is attributed to the fact that SAECG, instead of EP study was used for screening and therefore also resulted in inclusion of lower risk patients. Furthermore, the utility of CABG is thought to be a confounding factor as it is likely to improve overall prognosis. In the other trials, where VT/VF was documented or screened using EP study, which is considered to be an accurate screening tool in patients with underlying coronary artery disease (CAD), ICD was shown to be the best therapy. The most recently released trial, MUSTT, was significant in the fact that ICD therapy was even better than EP-guided therapy (Figure 2-1). Furthermore, in this trial, patients were prescribed drug therapy according to the current standard, including the use of beta blocker and ACE-inhibitor equally in both ICD and drug arms.

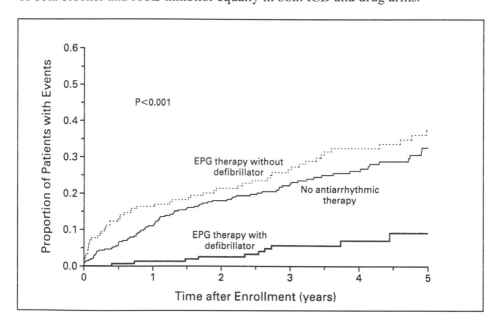

Figure 2-1. Estimates of the rates of cardiac arrest or death from arrhythmia. The P value refers to comparisons between EP-guided (EPG) therapy with ICD vs without ICD and EPG therapy with ICD vs no antiarrhythmic therapy, denoting superiority of ICD therapy to others (Ref 27).

Current Ongoing Trials

The recently completed clinical trials showed that in the management of patients with a history of VT/VF and patients with underlying ischemic cardiomyopathy considered to be at high risk for sudden death, ICD has become the overwhelming choice of therapy. ICD therapy is also assumed to be the best therapy for high-risk patients with underlying non-ischemic cardiomyopathy, although no data are yet available on this subset of patients. The SCD Heft (Sudden Cardiac Death, Heart Failure Trial), that enrolls ischemic and non-ischemic cardiomyopathy patients with Class II or III heart failure and low LVEF (<35%) to either receive ICD or placebo, will test the hypothesis that ICD lowers mortality in these patients.[36-38] It expects enrollment of 2500 patients. In this trial, EPS is not used as a stratification test. Other studies specifically enroll non-ischemic cardiomyopathy patients, such as the Defibrillators in Non-Ischemic Cardiomyopathy Treatment Evaluation (DEFINITE) trial, which expects to enroll over 440 patients to receive either ICD or no therapy and the German Dilated Cardiomyopathy Study (GDCMS). Other ongoing trials involving ischemic cardiomyopathy patients are also focusing in those with potential substrates without relying on electrophysiology study. Thus, MADIT II selects its patient enrollment based only on underlying LV dysfunction from ischemic heart disease, regardless of the arrhythmia history. The Defibrillator in Acute Myocardial Infarction Trial (DINAMIT) selects patients based on recent MI, low EF (of < 35%) and abnormal heart rate variability. The selection of these enrollment criteria is based on the overwhelming data from many controlled and uncontrolled studies that showed the underlying LV function as the strongest predictor of mortality and total outcome. Another ongoing trial, the Beta-blocker Strategy plus Implantable Cardioverter-Defibrillator Trial (BEST-ICD), however, assesses the role of antiarrhythmic drug or ICD versus no therapy, similar to MUSTT.

> **The results of ongoing trials will be important in helping clinician identify patients at risk and in guiding therapy for VT/VF prevention in a broader scope of patient population**

Thus, ongoing trials address the utility of ICD therapy in the broader scope of patients at risk. Furthermore, it will eliminate the utility of EPS, which has not been uniformly useful in all subsets of patients at risk. In fact, as the MUSTT study showed, EP-guided therapy with antiarrhythmic drugs was not beneficial. In that study, only ICD therapy was found to lower sudden death and total mortality. While such new and surprising findings could not be easily explained, they underscore the importance of a reliable therapy such as the ICD. At the same time, it poses a dilemma in the selection of risk stratification. Thus, the utility of other risk stratification, such as heart rate variability and T-wave alternans, is also being assessed.

- Data from completed large, randomized clinical trials on the use of ICD for secondary prevention of VT/VF (AVID, CIDS, CASH) have been nearly uniform in showing the superiority of ICD therapy over drug therapy in reducing sudden death and overall mortality.
- Data from completed clinical ICD trials for primary prevention (MADIT and MUSTT) have also showed superiority of ICD therapy over drug therapy. In the CABG-Patch study, which included revascularization therapy, there was no advantage of ICD therapy.
- The result of ongoing trials, mostly not utilizing EPS for stratification, would be useful in a broader scope of patients.

Current Practice Guidelines

The favorable data on ICD therapy, coupled with its rapid technological advances and improvements have resulted in the proliferation of ICD use over the past few years from just over 10,000 implants in the US in 1995 to over 50,000 in 1998, with a projective growth of 30-40% per year.[36,38-43]

The most current American College of Cardiology/American Heart Association (ACC/AHA) guidelines for ICD implantation was published in 1998 [44]. These recommendation have taken into account some of the data from clinical trials as well as smaller studies involving less well-defined population of patient at risk, such as those with long QT, hypertrophic cardiomyopathy and idiopathic VT/VF. These indications can be summarized as follows:

Class I Indications

(Conditions for which there is evidence and/or general agreement that a given procedure or treatment is beneficial, useful, and effective)

1. Cardiac arrest due to VF or VT not due to a transient or reversible cause.
2. Spontaneous sustained VT.
3. Syncope of undetermined origin with clinically relevant, hemodynamically significant sustained VT or VF induced at electrophysiological study when drug therapy is ineffective, not tolerated, or not preferred.
4. Nonsustained VT with coronary disease, prior MI, LV dysfunction, and inducible VF or sustained VT at electrophysiological study that is not suppressible by a Class I antiarrhythmic drug.

Class II-a Indications

(Conditions for which there is conflicting evidence/or a divergence of opinion about the usefulness/efficacy of a procedure or treatment and weight of evidence/opinion is in favor of usefulness/efficacy). For ICD, none is listed.

Class II-b Indications

(Conditions for which there is conflicting evidence/or a divergence of opinion about the usefulness/efficacy of a procedure or treatment and usefulness/efficacy is less well established by evidence/opinion)

1. Cardiac arrest presumed to be due to VF when electrophysiological testing is precluded by other medical conditions.
2. Severe symptoms attributable to sustained ventricular tachyarrhythmias while awaiting cardiac transplantation.
3. Familial or inherited conditions with a high risk for life-threatening ventricular tachyarrhythmias such as long QT syndrome or hypertrophic cardiomyopathy.
4. Nonsustained VT with coronary artery disease, prior MI, and LV dysfunction, and inducible sustained VT or VF at EP study.
5. Recurrent syncope of undetermined etiology in the presence of ventricular dysfunction and inducible ventricular arrhythmias at EP study when other causes of syncope have been excluded.

Class III Indications

(Conditions for which there is evidence and/or general agreement that a procedure/treatment is not useful/effective and in some cases may be harmful):

1. Syncope of undetermined cause in a patient without inducible ventricular tachyarrhythmias.
2. Incessant VT or VF.
3. VF or VT resulting from arrhythmias amenable to surgical or catheter ablation; for example, atrial arrhythmias associated with the Wolff-Parkinson-White syndrome, right ventricular outflow tract VT, idiopathic left ventricular tachycardia, or fascicular VT.
4. Ventricular tachyarrhythmias due to a transient or reversible disorder (e.g., acute MI, electrolyte imbalance, drugs, trauma).
5. Significant psychiatric illnesses that may be aggravated by device implantation or may preclude systematic follow-up.
6. Terminal illnesses with a projected life expectancy < 6 months
7. Patients with coronary artery disease with LV dysfunction and prolonged QRS duration in the absence of spontaneous or inducible sustained or nonsustained VT who are undergoing coronary artery bypass surgery.
8. NYHA Class IV drug-refractory congestive heart failure patients who are not candidates for cardiac transplantation.

> **Most recent guidelines incorporate data from large secondary and primary prevention trials and also allow physicians to use their clinical judgment in prescribing ICD**

Thus, in general, the latest guidelines classify those patients with cardiac arrest or sustained VT/VF, similar to those enrolled in the randomized trials for secondary prevention therapy, and patients who are considered at risk, similar to those enrolled in the randomized trials for primary prevention as definite candidates for ICD therapy. In the absence of large-scale clinical trials, other patients who are generally also considered to be at risk would have class II indication.

Some other clinical situations, which would not fall under the general indications of either class I or II, still may deserve individualized clinical decision. In some circumstances, even when there is a reversible cause, it would not be clinically reasonable to expect that such causes will not recur. For example, VT/VF that was associated with mild-to-moderate electrolyte imbalance is, in theory preventable. However, some patients maybe chronically at risk for having recurrences of electrolyte disorders such as patients with chronic renal insufficiency, idiopathic hypokalemia or hyperkalemia, and nutritional deficiency or disorders. Thus, the overall therapy, while mainly aimed at maintaining balanced electrolyte and metabolic status, may include an ICD.

In the example given below (Figure 2-2), recurrent polymorphic VT degenerated into rapid ventricular flutter, which, based on the patient's history, would have resulted in another cardiac arrest. The ICD was life saving, although the patient received multiple shocks from the repetitive nature of the polymorphic VT. Correction of her electrolyte imbalance was also necessary subsequently.

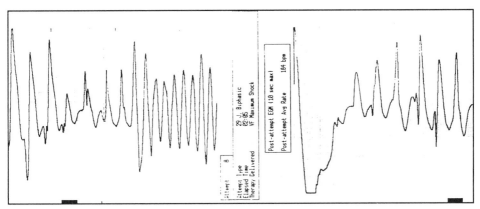

Figure 2-2. A recording from a patient with recurrent electrolyte imbalance from nutritional disorder. The tracing showed polymorphic VT that degenerated into ventricular flutter, which was successfully terminated by the ICD shock. The patient continued to suffer from recurrent polymorphic VT that required correction of her electrolyte imbalance.

Expanding Indications

It is not surprising that ICD therapy is gaining acceptance as the primary treatment for sudden death prevention. In many instances, drug therapy is not effective or not tolerated and therefore, ICD therapy is indicated in the majority of cases of primary and secondary prevention of VT/VF. Based on data from the most recently completed trial, MUSTT, ICD would be preferred over drug therapy because patients who were treated with drugs that were predicted to be effective by EP study still suffered a high recurrence of sudden death and had a high mortality rate. These data are contradictory to the general assumption and to data from prior, uncontrolled and nonrandomized clinical studies on the usefulness of EP study in selecting antiarrhythmic drug. Such a striking difference in clinical findings does not only highlight the relative weakness in small, uncontrolled studies, but also underscores the complexity of the clinical entity. The EP study may only be useful in elucidating one aspect of ventricular tachyarrhythmia. The disease entity is likely to be a complex, heterogeneous process that may be indeed best treated with a device that is capable of terminating tachyarrhythmia and preventing bradyarrhythmia. The possibility that antiarrhythmic drug therapy in itself may carry an inherent mortality risk is also of concern. With this particular issue in mind, clinicians would likely choose ICD as the more favorable therapy overall, regardless of the EP data, presenting arrhythmia, or underlying heart disease.[36,38,39,42,43,45-49]

In other, less well known situations, such as hypertrophic or idiopathic dilated cardiomyopathy, right ventricular dysplasia, long-QT syndrome, and other idiopathic ventricular tachyarrhythmia syndromes for which only minimal clinical data is available, ICD would also likely to be the therapy of choice.[50] For these clinical situations, large, well-controlled studies are not likely to occur, and the efficacy of antiarrhythmic drug is not known. Recently, the data from 128 patients with hypertrophic cardiomyopathy were released indicating the usefulness of ICD in this group.[51] The retrospective multi center study analyzed the incidence of ICD therapy in HCM patients who received the device for secondary (34%) and primary (66%) prevention. Appropriate device discharges occurred in both groups, in 44% of those with a history of sudden death and in 12% of those without, at a rate of 11% per year and 5% per year, respectively. Of the patients receiving appropriate therapy, 52%were on antiarrhythmic drugs (amiodarone, sotalol, or disopyramide). While this study does not provide definitive guidelines for the role of ICD in this patient population, it underscores the notion that sudden death is indeed caused by ventricular tachyarrhythmia and that the commonly used drugs such as amiodarone and sotalol have limited efficacy.

ICD is also likely to have a significant role in the management of patients with idiopathic cardiomyopathy. It this disease entity, it is clear that EP study is less useful. Furthermore, the disease process is progressive and carries a significant risk for both tachycardia and bradycardia-related morbidity and mortality, for which an ICD would be preferable over antiarrhythmic drug. The

SCD Heft Trial enrolls patients with ischemic and non-ischemic cardiomyopathy and randomizes them to one of three arms of treatment: ICD, empiric amiodarone, or non-specific antiarrhythmic therapy. This trial is particularly useful in identifying the potential utility of ICD in idiopathic cardiomyopathy patients.

The role of ICD in cardiomyopathy patients in general may also be expanding with the addition of biventricular pacing (see below). In cardiomyopathy patients with non-synchronous ventricular contraction due to delayed left ventricular conduction, ventricular synchronization with biventricular pacing has been shown to improve the status of congestive heart failure and functional class and the measured left ventricular ejection fraction.

Indications for Dual-Chamber ICD

As the use of ICD with dual-chamber pacing features is increasing, there is yet a formal guidelines for its indication. The dual-chamber ICD has advantages over the single chamber in many aspects that are beyond the advantages of dual-chamber pacemaker over single-chamber pacemaker. In addition to providing a more physiologic pacing for the patients requiring bradycardia support, the dual-chamber sensing capability would provide a much more discriminatory feature in differentiating VT from supraventricular arrhythmias.

ICD recipient patients who require bradycardia support also typically those in whom dual-chamber pacing would be clinically useful. In general, the patients are younger and more active. In addition, a significant subset of such patients has significant left ventricular dysfunction in which case dual-chamber pacing would be generally considered more advantageous. In addition to those considerations, the dual-chamber sensing discriminatory feature provides such a significant added advantage that the dual-chamber ICD is quite liberally prescribed. Thus, dual-chamber ICD is preferred over single-chamber in a significant majority of patients.

Thus, at the present time, the decision of for choosing dual-chamber ICD is based on several clinical factors that can be summarized as below:

1. Patients with traditional requirements for pacing for bradycardia support, such as symptomatic sinus node dysfunction and symptomatic paroxysmal or permanent atrioventricular block.
2. Patients who are showing early signs of sinus node dysfunction and conduction abnormality that are expected to worsen because of the need for antiarrhythmic drug therapy in addition to the ICD.
3. Patients who may benefit from dual-chamber arrhythmia discrimination features, such as patients with atrial tachyarrhythmias.

> - Guidelines for indication for ICD therapy are largely derived from data of recently completed large randomized clinical trials. Class I indications include patients who have had sudden death or sustained VT/VF not due to reversible causes (AVID/CIDS/CASH patients), and patients who are considered at risk (MADIT/MUSTT patients).
> - Other conditions that would probably pose high risk, such as IDCM, HCM, congenital Long-QT syndrome, Brugada syndrome and other idiopathic VF are within class II indications.
> - Indications for dual-chamber ICD have not been outlined. Current clinical practice has included patients who would benefit from the more physiologic dual-chamber bradycardia pacing as well as those in whom dual-chamber arrhythmia discriminatory features would be helpful.

Economical Impact of ICD Usage

One of the most concerning factor in the proliferation of ICD usage is, probably, its cost. The device costs significantly more than the pacemaker and despite its broader application and greater utility, the cost of the unit alone remains typically over U.S. $ 20,000.00. With the added costs of hospitalization and other associated procedures, the "price" for ICD implantation would typically be over $ 50,000.00. However, if the clinical benefit is considered into the equation of cost analysis, the cost of ICD therapy may compare favorably to other common cardiovascular treatments. Calculations of incremental cost of ICD over conventional antiarrhythmic drug therapy per Life-Year Saved (LYS) are, in general, within the $ 20,000.00 to $ 40,000.00 range[52-55], which is similar to the incremental cost of other common cardiovascular procedures, such as single-vessel coronary stenting, which was calculated at $ 31,244.[56] In fact, The "Dutch Study" reported a cost saving (rather than cost increment), but the comparison might not be applicable to today's standard of practice because the study utilized a high number of antiarrhythmic drug testing.[18] Of note, the cost analysis from AVID study showed a very high incremental cost, indicating that ICD therapy may not be cost effective (Table 2-2).

It would be important to keep in mind that cost analysis studies have many limitations. One important limitation is the constantly changing method in medical practice. Advancing technology, such as the transition from epicardial system to transvenous approach would significantly reduce hospitalization period and, consequently, the cost of implantation. Furthermore, increasing familiarity with the safety and efficacy of the device will probably result in lower rate of Emergency Room visits and re-hospitalizations. It should be noted that many of the studies analyzed ICD implantation in the era of epicardial implantation.[52,53,55] A review of databases of Medicare beneficiaries and California hospitals showed that with the initial change to the transvenous method in the early 1990s have shortened the length of stay for ICD implantation from an average of 27.4 days in 1987 to 10.8 days in 1995.[59] In this review, however, it was noted that hospital re-admissions were very frequent and showed little change.

Table 2-2. Incremental Cost per Life Year Saved

Study/Source	ICD System	Incremental Cost
Wever et al[18]	Epi- & endocardial	- $ 11,315 (net)
MADIT[54]	Endocardial (4yr battery life)	$ 28,751
	(if > 4yr battery life)	$ 13,311
Kuppermann et al[57]	Epicardial (4yr battery life)	$ 32,910
Kupersmith et al[52]	Epicardial (4yr battery life)	$ 36,257
Larsen et al[53]	Epicardial (2yr battery life)	$ 45,922
	(if 8yr battery life)	$ 24,219
Owens et al[55]	Endocardial (4yr battery life)	$ 57,502
AVID[58]	Endocardial (4yr battery life)	$ 114,917

It should also be noted that the studies cited above included ICD with shorter battery life.[54] Newer battery with greater longevity would prolong the time between implantation and therefore would be expected to reduce the overall cost of device therapy. Such sub-analysis was performed in two of the studies using devices with longer battery life. Other features, such as automatic capacitor reformation may also contribute in reducing cost by reducing the need for frequent outpatient visits.

On the other hand, it should be realized that there are other, "hidden" cost of any disease entity and its therapeutic approach. The above analyses only addressed the actual cost involved in the implementation of the treatment. There are other methods of analysis that could not be easily tracked such as the loss of income or productivity and the change in quality-of-life. Thus, cost analysis would be quite different from the patient and society point of view. In the case of ICD, such cost can be quite high when the patient becomes affected by the fear of shock and the stigma of having an artificial device or, on the contrary, quite low when the patient's confidence in his/her future prognosis is improved. In order to make an overall conclusion, all consideration must be included.

> **Although the price of the unit is relatively high, ICD therapy may prove to be cost effective if its life saving benefits are considered; however, so far there has not been a comprehensive analysis of this complex cost issue and therefore, clinicians should use their judgment in prescribing this therapy**

In summary, cost estimation and analysis is a complex issue and data from such analysis must be interpreted with great caution because there are too many variables involved. In general, it appears that ICD therapy may not turn out to be very cost effective unless the price of the unit decreases and until we have better methods of identifying patients who will receive a large treatment benefit.

- Economical impact of ICD therapy is an important consideration because the price of the unit and system is still quite high and is not likely to decline in the near future.
- If compared with the cost of other commonly utilized medical and surgical therapy (such as single-vessel coronary stenting), the cost of ICD therapy per Life-Year Saved is within reasonable range of $ 20,000 to $ 40,000.
- Analysis of the cost of ICD therapy is complex and influenced by many factors. While several factors (such as surgical, hospitalization, and ICD longevity) are discrete can be analyzed, other are difficult to quantify. Some cost-saving potential of the therapy (such as reduced hospitalization) may not manifest as predicted.

References

1. Mower MM and Nisam S. AICD indications (patient selection): past, present and future. Pacing Clin Electrophysiol, 1988;**11**(11 Pt 2):2064-2070.
2. Wilber DJ, Garan H, and Ruskin JN. Electrophysiologic testing in survivors of cardiac arrest. Circulation, 1987;**75**(4 Pt 2):III146-153.
3. Morady F, Scheinman MM, Hess DS, et al. Electrophysiologic testing in the management of survivors of out-of- hospital cardiac arrest. Am J Cardiol, 1983;**51**(1):85-89.
4. Swerdlow CD, Winkle RA, and Mason JW. Determinants of survival in patients with ventricular tachyarrhythmias. N Engl J Med, 1983;**308**(24):1436-1442.
5. Liem LB and Swerdlow CD. Value of electropharmacologic testing in idiopathic dilated cardiomyopathy and sustained ventricular tachyarrhythmias. Am J Cardiol, 1988;**62**(9):611-616.
6. Guiraudon G, Fontaine G, Frank R, et al. [Encircling endocardial ventriculotomy in the treatment of recurrent ventricular tachycardia after myocardial infarction]. Arch Mal Coeur Vaiss, 1982;**75**(9):1013-1021.
7. Klein H, Frank G, Werner PC, et al. [Results of electrophysiologically guided surgery in ventricular tachycardia]. G Ital Cardiol, 1983;**13**(4):318-322.
8. Vigano M, Martinelli L, Salerno JA, et al. Ventricular tachycardia in post-myocardial infarction patients. Results of surgical therapy. Eur Heart J, 1986;**7 Suppl A**:165-168.
9. Swerdlow CD, Mason JW, Stinson EB, et al. Results of operations for ventricular tachycardia in 105 patients. J Thorac Cardiovasc Surg, 1986;**92**(1):105-113.
10. Nath S, Haines DE, Kron IL, et al. The long-term outcome of visually directed subendocardial resection in patients without inducible or mappable ventricular tachycardia at the time of surgery. J Cardiovasc Electrophysiol, 1994;**5**(5):399-407.
11. Lehmann MH, Steinman RT, Schuger CD, et al. The automatic implantable cardioverter defibrillator as antiarrhythmic treatment modality of choice for survivors of cardiac arrest unrelated to acute myocardial infarction. Am J Cardiol, 1988;**62**(10 Pt 1):803-805.

12. Mirowski M, Reid PR, Winkle RA, et al. Mortality in patients with implanted automatic defibrillators. Ann Intern Med, 1983;98(5 Pt 1):585-588.

13. Mirowski M, Reid PR, Mower MM, et al. Clinical performance of the implantable cardioverter-defibrillator. Pacing Clin Electrophysiol, 1984;7(6 Pt 2):1345-1350.

14. Winkle RA, Mead RH, Ruder MA, et al. Long-term outcome with the automatic implantable cardioverter- defibrillator. J Am Coll Cardiol, 1989;13(6):1353-1361.

15. Fogoros RN, Elson JJ, Bonnet CA, et al. Efficacy of the automatic implantable cardioverter-defibrillator in prolonging survival in patients with severe underlying cardiac disease. J Am Coll Cardiol, 1990;16(2):381-386.

16. Cohen TJ, Reid PR, Mower MM, et al. The automatic implantable cardioverter-defibrillator. Long-term clinical experience and outcome at a hospital without an open-heart surgery program. Arch Intern Med, 1992;152(1):65-69.

17. O'Brien BJ, Buxton MJ, and Rushby JA. Cost effectiveness of the implantable cardioverter defibrillator: a preliminary analysis. Br Heart J, 1992;68(2):241-245.

18. Wever EF, Hauer RN, Schrijvers G, et al. Cost-effectiveness of implantable defibrillator as first-choice therapy versus electrophysiologically guided, tiered strategy in postinfarct sudden death survivors. A randomized study [see comments]. Circulation, 1996;93(3):489-496.

19. Moss AJ, Hall WJ, Cannom DS, et al. Improved survival with an implanted defibrillator in patients with coronary disease at high risk for ventricular arrhythmia. Multicenter Automatic Defibrillator Implantation Trial Investigators [see comments]. N Engl J Med, 1996;335(26):1933-1940.

20. A comparison of antiarrhythmic-drug therapy with implantable defibrillators in patients resuscitated from near-fatal ventricular arrhythmias. The Antiarrhythmics versus Implantable Defibrillators (AVID) Investigators [see comments]. N Engl J Med, 1997;337(22):1576-1583.

21. Siebels J and Kuck KH. Implantable cardioverter defibrillator compared with antiarrhythmic drug treatment in cardiac arrest survivors (the Cardiac Arrest Study Hamburg). Am Heart J, 1994;127(4 Pt 2):1139-1144.

22. Bigger JT, Jr. Prophylactic use of implanted cardiac defibrillators in patients at high risk for ventricular arrhythmias after coronary-artery bypass graft surgery. Coronary Artery Bypass Graft (CABG) Patch Trial Investigators [see comments]. N Engl J Med, 1997;337(22):1569-1575.

23. Connolly SJ, Gent M, Roberts RS, et al. Canadian Implantable Defibrillator Study (CIDS): study design and organization. CIDS Co-Investigators. Am J Cardiol, 1993;72(16):103F-108F.

24. Connolly S. Late Breaking Trials. Presented before ACC 47th Annual Scientific Session, March 30, 1998, 1998.

25. Kuck K. Late Breaking Trials. Presented before ACC 47th Annual Scientific Session, March 30, 1998, 1998.

26. Buxton AE. Ongoing risk stratification trials: the primary prevention of sudden death. Control Clin Trials, 1996;17(3 Suppl):47S-51S.

27. Buxton AE, Lee KL, Fisher JD, et al. A randomized study of the prevention of sudden death in patients with coronary artery disease. Multicenter Unsustained Tachycardia Trial Investigators. N Engl J Med, 1999;341(25):1882-1890.

28. Antiarrhythmics Versus Implantable Defibrillators (AVID)--rationale, design, and methods. Am J Cardiol, 1995;75(7):470-475.

29. The Coronary Artery Bypass Graft (CABG) Patch Trial. The CABG Patch Trial Investigators and Coordinators. Prog Cardiovasc Dis, 1993;36(2):97-114.

30. Bigger JT, Jr., Whang W, Rottman JN, et al. Mechanisms of death in the CABG Patch trial: a randomized trial of implantable cardiac defibrillator prophylaxis in patients at high risk of death after coronary artery bypass graft surgery. Circulation, 1999;99(11):1416-1421.

31. Curtis AB, Cannom DS, Bigger JT, Jr., et al. Baseline characteristics of patients in the coronary artery bypass graft (CABG) Patch Trial. Am Heart J, 1997;134(5 Pt 1):787-798.

32. Spotnitz HM, Herre JM, Raza ST, et al. Effect of implantable cardioverter-defibrillator implantation on surgical morbidity in the CABG Patch Trial. Surgical Investigators of the Coronary Artery Bypass Graft Patch Trial. Circulation, 1998;98(19 Suppl):II77-80.

33. Moss AJ. Background, outcome, and clinical implications of the Multicenter Automatic Defibrillator Implantation Trial (MADIT) [see comments]. Am J Cardiol, 1997;80(5B):28F-32F.

34. Akiyama T. Ventricular arrhythmias and sudden cardiac death: an insight from recent multicenter randomized clinical trials. Keio J Med, 1996;45(4):313-317.

35. Arenal Maiz A. [Prevention of sudden death after myocardial infarction: should the "MADIT" strategy be generally applied? Arguments against]. Rev Esp Cardiol, 1997;50(7):464-466.

36. Klein H, Auricchio A, Reek S, et al. New primary prevention trials of sudden cardiac death in patients with left ventricular dysfunction: SCD-HEFT and MADIT-II. Am J Cardiol, 1999;83(5B):91D-97D.

37.   Singh SN and Fletcher RD. Class III drugs and congestive heart failure: focus on the congestive heart failure-survival trial of antiarrhythmic therapy. Am J Cardiol, 1999;**84**(9A):103R-108R.

38.   Cannom DS. Other Primary Prevention Trials-What Is Clinically And Economically Necessary? J Interv Card Electrophysiol, 2000;**4 Suppl 1**:109-115.

39.   Higgins SL. Impact of the Multicenter Automatic Defibrillator Implantation Trial on implantable cardioverter defibrillator indication trends. Am J Cardiol, 1999;**83**(5B):79D-82D.

40.   Higgins SL, Williams SK, Pak JP, et al. Indications for implantation of a dual-chamber pacemaker combined with an implantable cardioverter-defibrillator. Am J Cardiol, 1998;**81**(11):1360-1362.

41.   Klein H and Trappe HJ. Implantable cardioverter defibrillator therapy: indications and decision making in patients with coronary artery disease. Pacing Clin Electrophysiol, 1992;**15**(4 Pt 3):610-615.

42.   Capucci A, Aschieri D, and Villani GQ. The Role of EP-Guided Therapy in Ventricular Arrhythmias: Beta- Blockers, Sotalol, and ICD's. J Interv Card Electrophysiol, 2000;**4 Suppl 1**:57-63.

43.   D Bc and Breithardt G. Evaluating AVID, CASH, CIDS, CABG-Patch & MADIT: Are They Concordant? J Interv Card Electrophysiol, 2000;**4 Suppl 1**:103-108.

44.   Gregoratos G, Cheitlin MD, Conill A, et al. ACC/AHA guidelines for implantation of cardiac pacemakers and antiarrhythmia devices: a report of the American College of Cardiology/American Heart Association Task Force on Practice Guidelines (Committee on Pacemaker Implantation). J Am Coll Cardiol, 1998;**31**(5):1175-1209.

45.   Hohnloser SH. Implantable devices versus antiarrhythmic drug therapy in recurrent ventricular tachycardia and ventricular fibrillation. Am J Cardiol, 1999;**84**(9A):56R-62R.

46.   Domanski MJ, Sakseena S, Epstein AE, et al. Relative effectiveness of the implantable cardioverter-defibrillator and antiarrhythmic drugs in patients with varying degrees of left ventricular dysfunction who have survived malignant ventricular arrhythmias. AVID Investigators. Antiarrhythmics Versus Implantable Defibrillators [see comments]. J Am Coll Cardiol, 1999;**34**(4):1090-1095.

47.   Andrews NP, Fogel RI, Pelargonio G, et al. Implantable defibrillator event rates in patients with unexplained syncope and inducible sustained ventricular tachyarrhythmias: a comparison with patients known to have sustained ventricular tachycardia. J Am Coll Cardiol, 1999;**34**(7):2023-2030.

48.   Cappato R. Secondary prevention of sudden death: the Dutch Study, the Antiarrhythmics Versus Implantable Defibrillator Trial, the Cardiac Arrest Study Hamburg, and the Canadian Implantable Defibrillator Study. Am J Cardiol, 1999;**83**(5B):68D-73D.

49.   Schmidinger H. The implantable cardioverter defibrillator as a "bridge to transplant": a viable clinical strategy? Am J Cardiol, 1999;**83**(5B):151D-157D.

50.   Elliott PM, Sharma S, Varnava A, et al. Survival after cardiac arrest or sustained ventricular tachycardia in patients with hypertrophic cardiomyopathy. J Am Coll Cardiol, 1999;**33**(6):1596-1601.

51.   Maron BJ, Shen WK, Link MS, et al. Efficacy of implantable cardioverter-defibrillators for the prevention of sudden death in patients with hypertrophic cardiomyopathy [see comments]. N Engl J Med, 2000;**342**(6):365-373.

52.   Kupersmith J, Hogan A, Guerrero P, et al. Evaluating and improving the cost-effectiveness of the implantable cardioverter-defibrillator. Am Heart J, 1995;**130**(3 Pt 1):507-515.

53.   Larsen GC, Manolis AS, Sonnenberg FA, et al. Cost-effectiveness of the implantable cardioverter-defibrillator: effect of improved battery life and comparison with amiodarone therapy. J Am Coll Cardiol, 1992;**19**(6):1323-1334.

54.   Mushlin AI, Hall WJ, Zwanziger J, et al. The cost-effectiveness of automatic implantable cardiac defibrillators: results from MADIT. Multicenter Automatic Defibrillator Implantation Trial. Circulation, 1998;**97**(21):2129-2135.

55.   Owens DK, Sanders GD, Harris RA, et al. Cost-effectiveness of implantable cardioverter defibrillators relative to amiodarone for prevention of sudden cardiac death [see comments]. Ann Intern Med, 1997;**126**(1):1-12.

56.   Kupersmith J, Holmes-Rovner M, Hogan A, et al. Cost-effectiveness analysis in heart disease, Part III: Ischemia, congestive heart failure, and arrhythmias. Prog Cardiovasc Dis, 1995;**37**(5):307-346.

57.   Kuppermann M, Luce BR, McGovern B, et al. An analysis of the cost effectiveness of the implantable defibrillator. Circulation, 1990;**81**(1):91-100.

58.   Larsen G, McAnulty J, Hallstrom A, et al. Hospitalization charges in the Antiarrhythmics Versus Implantable Defibrillators (AVID) trial: the AVID economic analysis study. Circulation, 1997;**96**(8):I-77.

59.   Hlatky M, Saynina O, McDonald K, et al. Utilization and outcomes of the implantable cardioverter defibrillator, 1987-1995. (submitted for publication), 2000.

CHAPTER 3

DEVICE OPERATION

The Basic ICD

The basic concept of safe and effective therapy for VT/VF has been the goal of the ICD, even during its early developmental stages. Thus, the concept of measuring a drop in right ventricular pressure as a means of detecting VF was abandoned in favor of the more reliable electrical signal monitoring.[1] Similarly, the early intravascular system was replaced by an epicardial system because of stability and safety concerns with the early right ventricular lead prototypes. The first generation of ICD lead system, which included an epicardial patch and a superior vena cava coil functioning as both sensing and defibrillating electrodes, was also quickly revised. Using the large area of a patch and a coil as a sensing mechanism had caused frequent oversensing of P waves, T waves, and post shock ST-T waves. The sensing method using probability density function (PDF), which detects a tachyarrhythmia based on the fraction of time the signal spends between positive and negative amplitude thresholds that are close to the baseline, was excellent in detecting VF. However, regular, non-sinusoidal VT was not reliably detected and hence, rate detection was soon added (AID-B and AID-BR units).[2] It was later noted that sensing reliability was markedly improved with the use of separate epicardial sensing leads placed closely together. This, along with two epicardial patches constituted the most commonly used epicardial ICD lead system.

The basic ICD device was a unit with a fixed energy output of 30 joules and also a fixed VT detection rate cut-off at a value between 150 and 185 beats/minute. A PDF feature was available in some units but this form of sensing enhancement was rarely used because of its known potential problem with under-detection of VT. Obviously, the clinician must be aware of any clinical factors that may interfere with this simple algorithm. An important clinical assessment would be to affirm that the patient would not have a hemodynamically significant VT at a rate slower than the fixed detection rate. Similarly, it should be assessed whether the patient could have sinus tachycardia or atrial tachyarrhythmia with a ventricular rate exceeding the detection rate. The need for a separate, and compatible bradycardia device would also have to be considered.

Even with such shortcomings, the performance of the basic ICD unit was satisfactory in most instances. The system's safety and efficacy were reflected in the results of its first large clinical data.[3,4] Clinicians were not too concerned with the lack of practical features in these early devices. The respond was an overall appraisal of a therapy that was effective for patients with a serious arrhythmia, which was refractory to medical or surgical therapy. The clinicians' concern echoed the original inventor intention of designing a device that is safe and effective.

In its early development, ICD features were simplified as to optimize detection of both VF and VT

One important progress in ICD operational feature is the addition of pacing therapy. Pacing for bradycardia, in the form of simple ventricular demand (VVI) mode was added first (e.g. in Ventak P2 and P3 CPI units). Afterwards, antitachycardia pacing (ATP) feature was incorporated, along with tiered-therapy feature, thus allowing for separate therapy programming for VT and VF. With these therapy features, the ICD technology reached a new platform as it then provided a therapy for a broader spectrum of arrhythmia, although with a very basic bradycardia therapy component. The Ventak P was the first CPI unit to include these features. At that time, other pacemaker manufactures also produced ICD units with similar features. Ventritex (Sunnyvale, CA) introduced Cadence and Medtronic (Minneapolis, MN) introduced PCD (Pacemaker Cardioverter Defibrillator). Shortly thereafter, other models were also introduced; Guardian by Telectronics (Englewood, CO), Res-Q by Intermedics (Angleton, TX), and Siecure by Siemens Pacesetter (Sylmar, CA). The Ventritex unit, Cadence was the first to incorporate biphasic waveform. Because of its superiority, biphasic waveform was soon incorporated in other ICD models, such as Ventak P2 and PRx II (CPI), PCD 7219 (Medtronic), and Res-Q (Intermedics).

In addition to their more versatile operational scope, these third generation units were also slightly smaller than the early, first generation units and some, like the Medtronic PCD 7219, which was 83 ml in volume and weighing 136 grams, was small enough to be considered as suitable for pectoral implant. Naturally, the ICD system transformed from a thoracotomy to an endocardial system. In late 1980s, CPI tested the Endotak nonthoracotomy leads. At the same time or shortly thereafter, other manufacturers designed and began testing their own endocardial lead systems such as the Transvene by Medtronic, EnGuard by Telectronics, and similar ones by others. Initially, there were variations to the non-thoracotomy approach. The incorporation of additional electrodes, such as the coronary sinus lead as part of the Transvene system, and the subcutaneous patch or array electrodes, was necessary to achieve effective defibrillation. However, later, with the use of biphasic waveform, a system with a single right ventricular lead incorporating one or two coils and/or in combination with the generator as another electrode, provided sufficient margin of safety and became the standard approach.

Advancements in battery and capacitor technology allowed for the design of smaller generators and accordingly, subsequent development of ICD was aimed at the production of progressively smaller units; e.g. the CPI's Ventak Mini family, Medtronic's Jewel and Micro Jewel models, and Ventritex' Cadet. These smaller ICD generators were more suitable for pectoral implantation and further simplify the transvenous implantation method. At such a reduced size, these smaller units can be implanted with an approach virtually identical to permanent pacemaker implantation. Some models, such as the Ventritex units, also offer modified shapes and reduced thickness to further accommodate pectoral placement (Figure 3-1), while others continue to miniaturize while incorporating more features including dual-chamber functions, such as the Medtronic models (Figure 3-2).

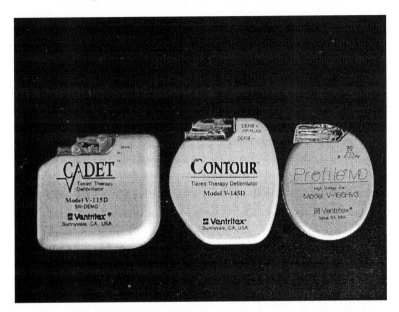

Figure 3-1. From left to right: The Ventritex Cadet (76 cc, 20.3 mm), Contour (57 cc, 15 mm), and Profile (34 cc, 11 mm)

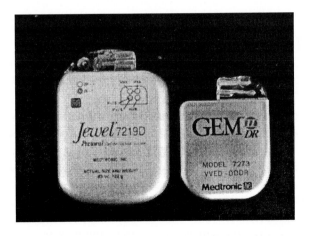

Figure 3-2. The Medtronic Jewel 7219D (83 cc, 18 mm) and GEM II DR (39 cc, 13.5 mm)

Occasionally, special consideration must be given to patients with a small pectoral area to avoid over-protrusion of the pocket and risk for erosion and infection and a submuscular implantation may be necessary in such a situation. In the majority of cases, however, a transvenous lead passage and a subcutaneous pocket would be the standard procedure.

The ICD progressed from a simple defibrillator to a device with a broader scope of antiarrhythmic therapy and a system that is simpler to implant
---

Throughout its progress, the ICD remains a very reliable and effective form of therapy because its core function as a defibrillator is maintained. The unit is always equipped with a sufficient amount of defibrillation capacity and a very sensitive sensing mechanism to detect VF. Its newer, additional features are implemented only for providing better energy delivery and arrhythmia discrimination with a high priority of preserving sensitivity of VF and VT detection. The concept of rapid, safe and optimal defibrillation takes precedence over all other functions.

- The first implantable defibrillators (AICD) had basic, non-programmable but reliable functions. Sensing was rate-base with PDF option, detection rate cut-off was fixed, and all therapies were high-energy shock at 30 or 35 joules.
- The second and third generations ICD added pacing and tier-therapy features but maintained the basic operation algorithm.
- Even with subsequent progress in miniaturizing the pulse generator, the ICD maintains its basic high sensitivity and safe therapy features.

Defibrillation Concept and Technology

Optimal Defibrillation Methods

It has been long known that ventricular fibrillation can be terminated by passing an electrical current at an adequate intensity for an adequate period of time.[5] Early experiment data indicated that there was possibly a simple dose response relationship for successful defibrillation, similar to the concept of cardiac pacing. Further notions from clinical experience in transthoracic and open-chest defibrillation that the energy required for defibrillation correlated with the size of the heart and the subject supported such hypothesis.[6-9] However, it was also recognized later that there were many aspects of defibrillation that defied the simple theory. A shock with excessive strength might fail to defibrillate and hence, the strength duration curve for effective defibrillation might not follow the conventional curve.[10] Also, the defibrillation threshold follows a sigmoidal relationship rather than a linear one.[11,12] Furthermore, success of defibrillation is unpredictable. A shock of certain strength may be effective in one occasion but fail at another attempt.

The concept of defibrillation can be better appreciated through the understanding the mechanism of fibrillation.[13] The critical mass concept of fibrillation provides a better explanation for the mechanism defibrillation.[14-16] The theory that fibrillation is initiated and sustained by continuous reentry of its wavelets is consistent with the concept that it requires a critical mass. This is supported by empirical observation that small hearts are difficult to fibrillate while large hearts are difficult to defibrillate. Thus, to be successful, a defibrillation shock must reduce the excitable volume of the heart to below this critical mass or, conversely, defibrillation must depolarize a critical volume or mass. If sufficient amount of the heart is depolarized by the defibrillating shock, there will not be enough excitable tissue to support the fibrillatory wavefront.

For a defibrillation shock to be effective, it must create sufficient potential (voltage) gradient and current density on throughout the applied area of the heart.[15,17,18] This concept is also important clinically because of the limitations present with the amount of energy that could be delivered by the defibrillator and because of the variation in current distribution in the heart and other parts of the body. The variation in current distribution in the various tissues is governed by several factors. One is the relative distant between the tissue and the electrode source of energy.[19] Another factor is the tissue resistivity, which is not only tissue specific, but is also anisotropic.[20-26] In the canine heart, for example, resistivity is three times higher across than along the muscle fibers. Yet another important factor, especially in the case of defibrillation is the electrical state of the tissue, as partially depolarized tissue requires a larger potential gradient than a fully repolarized one for the generation of a new action potential.[27-31] Of particular importance is the observation that these partially repolarized tissues exhibit partial depolarization when excited by a voltage gradient at above certain critical value. This value is different for different species and with different waveform. In dogs, it is about 6 V/cm with a 7 ms truncated monophasic waveform and about 4 V/cm for 5 ms biphasic waveform.[32-35] The degree of prolongation was noted to vary directly with the size of the stimulus and the time from the start of repolarization, such that a particular voltage gradient would prolong refractoriness in such a way that all cells would recover almost simultaneously.

Such prolongation of refractoriness promotes uniformity of tissue recovery and prevents propagation of any remaining activation front and reentry of post-shock repetitive responses that would otherwise cause re-fibrillation. Such repetitive responses may imitate VF but typically they occur with coupling intervals that are longer than the R-R intervals during VF (Figure 3-3). Repetitive responses after a shock is not uncommon and is probably generated by the shock itself but if the shock generates sufficient voltage gradient to cause a sufficient uniform prolongation of refractoriness, re-fibrillation would not occur.

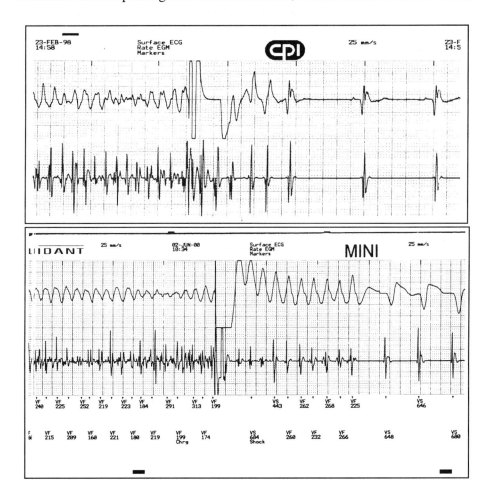

Figure 3-3. Two examples of repetitive responses after a shock that failed to re-initiate VF

Such factors are important to take into consideration if depolarization of a critical mass is necessary for successful defibrillation. The shock energy must be sufficient to not only distribute to the critical volume of myocardium but to create sufficient voltage gradient as to affect the critical volume and to depolarize them and extend their refractoriness simultaneously. Of clinical importance is the observation that the difference in potential gradient between the highest and the lowest sites can vary significantly, ranging from 4 to 1 in the case of transthoracic defibrillation to 20 to 1 in the case of epicardial or intracardiac defibrillation.[36,37] Thus, for the ICD, it would be necessary to create a voltage gradient of 80 to 120 V/cm in the nearest tissue. However, it is also known that a very high stimulus, such as those exceeding 200 V/cm, can create cellular damage by electroporation, a dielectric breakdown of the cellular membrane.[38-40] Thus, the "dose" of defibrillation must be high enough as to assure delivery of sufficient voltage gradient at the distant sites and capture of the critical volume of the myocardium, yet not too large as to cause cellular damage at the site near the electrodes.

> **Some concepts of effective defibrillation, such as the generation of sufficient voltage gradient and the depolarization of a critical mass are important not only to the design of ICD system but also to its implementation and implantation**

It is also noted that an unsuccessful defibrillation creates new activation front, which then encounters a partially refractory tissue and propagates reentry and initiate re-fibrillation. This is believed to be caused by a shock that is sufficient to alter the activation sequence of the critical volume of the myocardium but is too weak to prolong refractoriness and hence would give rise to new activation front and initiate re-fibrillation. This form of re-fibrillation is similar to the manner in which fibrillation is induced by a large stimulus given during the vulnerable period. The similarities in the initiation of fibrillation by the T-wave shock and the re-initiation of fibrillation by a failed defibrillation shock is the basis for "upper limit of vulnerability" hypothesis.[41,42] Experimentally it was found that a sufficiently strong shock would not initiate or re-initiate fibrillation no matter when it is delivered during the vulnerable period. The shock strength above which fibrillation is not induced is termed the upper limit of vulnerability. This is also important clinically because the defibrillation threshold can be estimated by this upper limit of vulnerability value.[43-46] It would be then easy to understand some of the inconsistency of the results of defibrillation when the shock strength applied is near this value. A slight influence of automaticity or metabolic environment may change this value and a shock that would otherwise be successful for defibrillation may re-initiate fibrillation and fail. Therefore, the defibrillation threshold is of a probabilistic nature rather than an all-or-none.

> **Depending on its strength, a shock may fibrillate or defibrillate the heart and therefore the "defibrillation threshold" can be estimated by measuring the upper limit of vulnerability**

As mentioned above, the defibrillation waveform of an ICD is critical in the delivery of an effective yet safe shock. In addition, there are the obvious technical limitations involved in the design of shock delivery from the small implantable units. For the implantable devices, the best waveform is the low tilt truncated pulse. Such a waveform is clinically beneficial because it avoids the delivery of unnecessarily high initial current, which may cause tissue damage and also limits the delivery of low strength current at the terminal portion, which is believed to cause re-initiation of fibrillation. From the technical point of view it is also advantageous because it requires lower initial energy delivery from the capacitor.

A single truncated waveform is called monophasic, the waveform that was utilized in all early models of ICDs. Modifications to this basic waveform were then tested in the search for a more effective energy delivery. Some of the variations that were tested were sequential, simultaneous and double pulses.[47-53] These modifications were indeed noted to have improved defibrillation capacity, but their application would require more complex defibrillation electrode configuration and, furthermore, the reduction in defibrillation energy requirement was not substantial.

The breakthrough of defibrillation delivery technology was the discovery of biphasic waveform.[54-57] With the biphasic waveform, where the first and second parts of the waveform are delivered with opposite polarities, it was found that the energy required for defibrillation is significantly reduced.[54,55] This was found to be due to the lower requirement for producing the extension of refractoriness in the partially repolarized cells.[30,33,58] It should be noted, however, that there are multiple factors influencing the beneficial effect of biphasic waveform. Early investigation showed that the optimal reduction in defibrillation threshold is noted only when the first pulse duration is at least equal to the second pulse duration; otherwise, an increase in defibrillation threshold may be produced.[54]

Another favorable feature of the biphasic waveform is its superiority over monophasic waveform in prolonged fibrillation. With fibrillation lasting up to 30 seconds, it was noted that while the defibrillation threshold of a monophasic waveform rises significantly, that of a biphasic waveform increases only slightly.[59] This is believed to be due to the ability of biphasic waveform to stimulate potassium-induced depolarized cells in addition to its superiority in prolonging refractoriness in partially repolarized tissues.[33,34,58,60]

> **Biphasic waveform lowers the energy requirement for defibrillation, which is instrumental in the progress and overall success in ICD therapy**

There has been significant amount of work in the search of optimal biphasic waveform, including the initial polarity, the total and individual pulse amplitude and duration, the degree of tilt, and other variables. Further research may still be necessary, as the data so far have been, in general, non-uniform and inconclusive. For example, several investigators have reported the benefit of using anodal ("reversed") polarity as the initial waveform[61-65] while the works of many others failed to show such benefit.[66-69] There has been also extensive research on the effect of the respective pulse duration on the DFT.[54,55,70-72] The early studies have shown, in general, the benefit of a longer first pulse. However, other variables may influence this parameter and insufficient data are available at this point.[72,73] Furthermore, This parameter is normally not programmable in ICD units, and therefore, would have limited clinical relevance in its clinical management.

One parameter that is closely related to the phase duration and directly influences it is the degree tilt. The tilt is the amount of voltage drop of the truncated waveform (Figure 3-4).

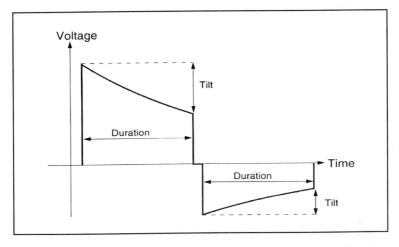

Figure 3-4. A diagram of a biphasic waveform with its components. The tilt is the amount of voltage drop at the truncation of the waveform (Reproduced with permission from Medtronic).

Many ICD units with biphasic waveform use a truncation after a 65% voltage drop (and is designated as a 65% tilt). With recent data showing the advantage of a lesser drop of 50% (which would also result in shorter phase duration) [74-80], some Medtronic ICD units (GEM models) utilize this value (Figure 3-5). Some ICD units (Ventritex ICD) offer programmable tilt.

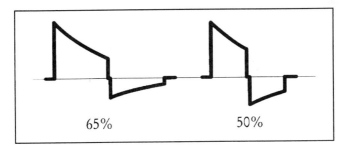

Figure 3-5. Comparison of 65% and 50% tilts

Overall, defibrillation with a biphasic waveform can be accomplished with an energy of approximately half of that required with a monophasic pulse. With its use, the success of ICD implantation has come close to 100%, even with the variable utility of the type of lead and ICD generator. However, the clinician is occasionally faced with a high DFT situation. In such a case, consideration should be made in terms of changing or varying programmable waveform parameters.

- The key components to successful defibrillation are the creation of sufficient voltage gradient and the depolarization of sufficient amount of tissue. These would ensure simultaneous depolarization of tissues of all states (including those that are already partially depolarized) and uniform prolongation of refractoriness to prevent re-fibrillation from new activation front.
- Defibrillation energy should not be too large or too concentrated as to cause cellular damage of tissue near the defibrillation electrode.
- The appropriate dose of defibrillation is closely related to the upper limit of vulnerability (ULV), the highest energy that could induce fibrillation when given in the vulnerable period of repolarization.
- Biphasic defibrillation pulse provides lower defibrillation threshold, probably by lowering the requirement for producing extension of repolarization in partially repolarized cells. All current ICD units use biphasic pulse for therapy. Monophasic pulse is still available in some units for use with T-wave shock.
- The degree of tilt of defibrillation pulse may also influence the efficacy of defibrillation

Defibrillation Electrodes and Leads

There have been numerous types of ICD defibrillation electrode and lead systems tested. Interestingly, one of the early prototype designs was already a single endovascular system. The lead was designed similar to a pacemaker lead system, with a right ventricular placement, and was intended to perform as both a shocking and sensing unit. However, these early endovascular models required a higher current, voltage, and energy for defibrillation than a transventricular system and therefore, subsequent prototypes were designed to include the use of one or more epicardial patches (Figure 3-6).

Various configurations of transventricular defibrillation systems were then tested, including the combinations incorporating epicardial, endocardial, and subcutaneous leads. In conjunction with these variations, various types of defibrillation pulses were also tested, including sequential and simultaneous pulses delivered through different sets of electrodes. These modified pulse delivery systems were noted to lower defibrillation energy requirements and therefore some were implemented in the design of various ICD models. The Medtronic units utilized the combination of right ventricular (RV) apical coil, superior vena caval (SVC) coil, and coronary sinus coil, as well as a subcutaneous patch. The Guidant-CPI units utilized the combination of RV/SVC coils with subcutaneous patch or array. In addition, both sequential and simultaneous pulses with polarity variations were tested using these electrode configurations.

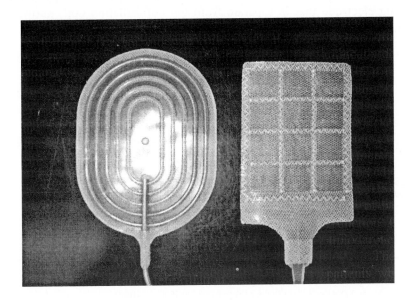

Figure 3-6. Epicardial patches made by Medtronic (left) and CPI (right)

With the advent of biphasic waveform, however, defibrillation energy requirement was significantly lowered, eliminating the need for multiple electrode combinations. Furthermore, the incorporation of the generator unit itself as an active defibrillation electrode also obviates the need for a subcutaneous patch. It is very unusual, nowadays, to have to include the various electrode combinations, unless one encounters a situation with a very high defibrillation threshold.

The integration of sensing and defibrillating functions using the same electrodes that was used in the early prototypes were found to have many disadvantages. A strong defibrillation shock would typically create sensing and pacing problems if applied through the same electrodes. Furthermore, the large electrode surface needed for defibrillation would not be ideal for sensing and pacing purposes. Hence subsequent electrode prototypes utilized separate systems for sensing and defibrillation. For epicardial system, the defibrillation electrodes usually comprised of small or large epicardial patches while the sensing electrodes are a pair of epicardial screw-in leads or a bipolar endocardial lead. In the subsequent system utilizing endocardial lead, the sensing and defibrillation electrodes would run through the same lead but positioned at different locations. Typically, the sensing/pacing electrodes would be positioned at the tip of the lead, similar to a pacing lead, while the defibrillation electrode(s) positioned proximally. In many leads (those manufactured by CPI and Ventritex), the proximal (anode) sense/pace electrode is combined into the distal defibrillation coil. This configuration is known as the "integrated bipolar sense/pace" type (Figure 3-7). In others (such as those manufactured by Medtronic and Biotronik), the sense/pace bipolar electrodes comprised of a tip and a ring electrode that is separate from the defibrillation coil, known as the "true bipolar system."

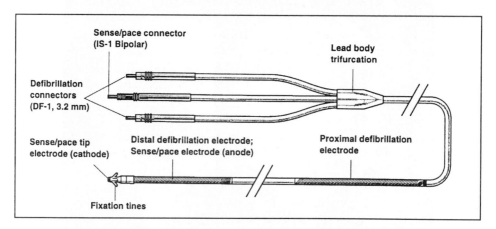

Figure 3-7. A schematic of a typical ICD lead with two defibrillation coils and an integrated bipolar pace/sense system (Reproduced with permission from St.Jude).

The term unipolar or bipolar is not commonly used to denote defibrillation pulse energy delivery because at times, multiple electrodes are involved. However, the concept can still be applied, but with less clinical relevant. For example, the simplest system using a single defibrillation coil as one electrode and the generator itself as the other resembles a unipolar pacing configuration, while one delivering the energy solely between two endocardial coils resembles the bipolar configuration. Of more clinical importance is the fact that, unlike pacemaker pulse delivery, defibrillation polarity can be reversed. In fact, some studies indicate that reversing polarity by using the distal defibrillation coil as the anode, may lower defibrillation threshold.[61-63,65,81] It should be noted that reversal of polarity does not uniformly reduce DFT and, in fact, some studies showed that it would not improve defibrillation success.[66-69]

> ICD electrode and lead system has evolved from one that comprised of multiple epicardial components to a single endocardial lead while maintaining separate high-integrity sensing and defibrillation function

In terms of electrode and lead material, many factors influenced its choice and engineering. Obviously, much of its progress is influenced by the knowledge obtained from the development of pacemaker technology. Materials used in lead construction must satisfy biocompatibility and biostability, and hence, those with known performance characteristics in pacemaker technology were the natural choices.[82-85] Investigations of any new material must include extensive biocompatibility performance testing in animals before human implants and would naturally take many years of development. Most defibrillation leads are, therefore, similar to their pacemaker counterparts. In particular, the insulation material of defibrillation lead closely resembles pacemaker leads, i.e. either silicone or polyurethane.[86-89]

Silicone rubber is suitable for lead insulation because it is a good flexible insulator that is biostable, biocompatible and inert. It consists of many components with specific properties that are mixed in certain combinations to provide the desired characteristics. In particular, the silica provides flexibility and tensile strength. One disadvantage is its lower resistance to tearing. To compensate for its lower tear strength, silicone leads are made slightly larger. Another distinct characteristic of the silicone lead is its higher coefficient of friction, causing them to be more likely to stick together. While this would not cause any problems with epicardial leads, which are mostly of silicone material, it could pose some technical challenge for endocardial placement, especially when multiple leads are involved. Silicone is used in all epicardial patches as these leads would benefit from the flexibility of this material and would not need to be very thin. Silicone is also used in the endocardial leads produced by Guidant-CPI manufacturer.

Polyurethane insulation material is the alternative to silicone and has been found to have similar characteristics in terms of biocompatibility.[82,83] It has higher tear strength then silicone and allows for smaller diameter leads.[90]. Furthermore, its low friction characteristic is an advantage in the case of a multiple endocardial lead placement.[83] However, this material may have lower biostability properties[87,88,90,91] and has been noted to have insulation failure, which is believed to be due to either environmental stress cracking or metal ion oxydation. Environmental stress produces cracking in this insulation material, typically at sharp bends or kinks or at a suture site. A higher degradation, for example, was noted with subclavian approach when compared to cephalic technique.[91] Metal ion oxydation is believed to occur from the interaction between hydrogen peroxide released from inflammatory cells and metal ions from defibrillator conductors. Other studies, however, showed similar stability between silicone and polyurethane leads.[92] Polyurethane is used in Medtronic endocardial leads.

> **ICD lead material is similar to that used in pacemaker technology and is likely to perform with similar advantages and disadvantages**

Past experience in pacemaker technology has also provided basic insight into the development of defibrillation electrode. Electrode materials must be highly conductive, as well as biostable and biocompatible with a low corrosive tendency. Titanium has been found to be suitable material for this purpose[93][94] and a titanium mesh is used for defibrillator patches made by Guidant-CPI and Telectronics manufacturers. Another suitable material for electrodes is platinum[95-100], which is non-corrosive and is highly conductive. By itself it is too soft, and therefore it is usually used with iridium as Pt/Ir alloy. Platinum-iridium had been used for catheter lead-mounted ring electrodes for pacemaker technology. For defibrillation leads, Pt/Ir is used in Medtronic and Ventritex patches, and endocardial defibrillation coils of Medtronic and Guidant-CPI manufacturers. Other, new suitable materials, such as carbon is also being investigated.[101-103]

Of also some clinical importance is the design of the defibrillation coil. In order to minimize voltage drop along the length of the defibrillation coil, a direct conductor is inserted in the Guidant-CPI models. This is believed to provide better defibrillation electrical field. However, the high voltage generated at the distal tip near the sensing electrode may cause post-shock sensing problems, especially in the integrated system.[104] The Medtronic coil is not equipped with such a conductor, and therefore provides lower voltage delivery at the distal end but, on the other hand, it is associated with less post-shock sensing abnormalities.

> **ICD electrode materials are also similar to those used in pacemaker systems and are subjected to similar wear and tear**

There are numerous other characteristics of the defibrillation lead that play some role in its performance, safety, and longevity. Many changes have been made for the purposes of improving sensing, pacing and defibrillation functions. Improvements in stability, durability, and size are also part of the development of the leads but many factors that influence these parameters may not be evident until longer experience with endocardial leads is achieved.

- To assure optimal energy delivery and to avoid tissue damage, defibrillation electrodes were designed as epicardial patches. In the transition to endocardial system, combination of multiple endovascular electrodes and subcutaneous patches/arrays were used. With the availability of efficient defibrillation with biphasic waveform, single endocardial lead against the pulse generator as the other electrode is sufficient.
- In some lead models, the defibrillation coil electrode is also used as one of the sensing electrode, known as the "integrated bipolar" system.
- The electrode material is either titanium (in some patches) or platinum/iridium alloy (in many endocardial leads).
- Silicone is used for insulation material for the defibrillation electrode patches. For the endocardial lead, both silicone and polyurethane are used, each for its specific advantages that were found to be useful in pacemaker technology.

Batteries and Capacitors

One clear difference between pacemaker and ICD technology is in the energy storage and delivery. The energy that an ICD must deliver is several orders in magnitude larger than that of a pacemaker. An ICD delivers, on the average, up to 30 joules of energy in a few milliseconds while a pacemaker typically delivers 1 to 10 microjoules.

In terms of battery material, a low resistance compound is more appropriate for ICDs because a high voltage must be maintained after delivery of a high current. The battery chemistry remains lithium based because this material offers advantageous inherent properties such as stability, high energy density, and fast discharge kinetics.[105] However, the standard lithium-iodine with high internal impedance that is ideal for pacemakers is not suitable for implantable defibrillators. For ICD, lithium-vanadium oxide and lithium-silver-vanadium oxide materials with lower impedance are more suitable.[106] Lowering internal resistance is also accomplished by using high anodal and cathodal surface areas and consequently, ICD battery is typically larger than its pacemaker counterpart.

Unlike a pacemaker, the ICD with a typical battery voltage of 3.2 V must deliver up to 750 V for defibrillation. This is accomplished mainly by utilizing capacitors. Capacitors are energy storage components and its storage capacity is dependent upon its material and volume. Typically, two or three capacitors connected in series are required. The addition of these capacitors that are typically large and their insulating materials is main the reason for the relatively large ICD unit.[107] Ongoing investigation on various capacitors and its characteristics has improved the understanding of their performance and are likely to result in further minimizing its size.[72,73,108,109]

> Unlike a pacemaker, an ICD must be able to deliver a high voltage over a short period of time; this is accomplished by using capacitors and batteries with lower impedance

Another method for facilitating the rapid delivery of high voltage is with the use of two batteries in series, which is used in some ICD models. With this configuration, charging to full capacity is accomplished a few seconds sooner than with the use of a single battery. However, this difference is typically small (in the order of two to three seconds) and in the interest of size, however, most new ICD models are equipped with a single battery. Thus, depending on the number of battery, at its beginning-of-life (BOL), an ICD may have a voltage of 6.4 or 3.2 volts.

A clinically important characteristic of currently used capacitors (of aluminum electrolytes) is the need for periodic charging (known as "reforming") because of slow dielectric deterioration. Otherwise, the time required to fully charge the capacitor could be excessively prolonged. In older ICD models, the capacitors must be reformed manually, requiring the patients to be seen in follow-up at frequent intervals of every two to three months. Most ICD models now have the capability of automatically reform the capacitors, which is nominally done every three or four month. This would obviate the need for frequent follow-up although the information would still need to be retrieved.

With time, the battery voltage drops and internal resistance increases. Both parameters, as well as the time to fully charge the capacitors are used to warn that the unit is near its end-of-life (EOL). Such elective replacement indicator (ERI) is usually set to allow several months before the unit reaches EOL and becomes nonfunctional.

> - ICD differs markedly from pacemaker in terms of energy storage and delivery.
> - Like pacemakers, ICD batteries are lithium-based because of its advantageous properties in terms of stability, high energy density and fast discharge kinetics. Unlike pacemakers, ICD batteries must have low impedance, which is accomplished by using lithium-vanadium or lithium-silver-vanadium material and by increasing the anodal and cathodal surface areas.
> - The BOL voltage of an ICD may be 3.2 V or 6.4 V, depending on whether one or two batteries are used, respectively.
> - To deliver up to 750 volts with the same 3.2-volts battery, ICD uses capacitors. Current capacitors using aluminum electrolytes undergo dielectric deterioration and require periodic charging.
> - The large battery surface and multiple capacitors comprise the bulk of the pulse generator volume.

The Defibrillation Threshold Concept

Clinical data have confirm early results of ICD studies that an internal defibrillation, even with using monophasic waveform, can be accomplished with an average of about 20 joules. Hence most devices were equipped with a maximum capacity of 30 joules. To accommodate situation with high DFT, some units with capability of delivering 35 joules or 40 joules were made available, in keeping with the general principle of providing an adequate margin of safety.

Analogous to the determination of capture threshold in the pacemaker technology, it would be desirable to measure the efficacy and reliability of defibrillation. Unlike the determination of pacing threshold, the measurement of defibrillation threshold (DFT) is more limited because, obviously, induction and defibrillation of VF can not be performed as liberally as with pacing. Furthermore, the DFT is not a precise measurement. It is influenced by many technical and clinical factors; many of which are still poorly understood. One clinical factor that was recognized early was the type and duration of VF.[110]

This study, however, compared DFT requirements for VF at various duration, including those at 30 and 35 second, which is not an atypical scenario for early ICD models such as the AID units. In considering later ICD models, it appeared that within the roam of their typical capacity, this factor has minimal clinical relevance.[111] It was noted that there was no significant increase in the DFT requirements between VF lasting 20 seconds and 10 seconds. Furthermore, these observations and concerns were noted with the use of monophasic waveform. With the use of biphasic waveform, the increase in DFT with longer VF duration is even less of a concern.[33,34,59,60,112]

The obtained value is certainly also influenced by the method and algorithm utilized. At best, the DFT is a statistical value and only an approximation of the true "threshold". Such estimation follows the sigmoidal probability curve, which means that the lower the energy required for defibrillation, the more the curve is parallel to a 100% efficacy. In clinical practice this means that if a very low energy is required for defibrillation, there is a greater consistency of that value, providing a higher degree of confidence that a shock at that level would be effective. Unfortunately, the sigmoidal curve also means that when the "DFT" is relatively high, at the steeper portion of the curve, there would be less consistency in the efficacy of such a shock in being successful at terminating VF. It can thus be appreciated that it would be desirable to measure the DFT as accurately as possible.

> **The defibrillation "threshold" is important parameter to know in order to program the device with sufficient margin of safety but, at best, this value can only be estimated because the relationship between successful defibrillation and shock energy is a sigmoidal probability curve**

Various methods have been used for DFT measurement.[12,113-117] The two common methods are the step-down method and the binary method. In the step-down method, DFT testing is started at a high-energy value, such as 20 joules, and is carried on with a progressively lower value until failure. This method would tend to overestimate the DFT. Alternatively, a step-up method can be used, starting with a low value. This method would underestimate the true DFT. With the binary method, the testing is started at a mid-range value, such as 12 or 15 joules, and is carried on to either a higher or lower value depending on its success or failure and at a progressively lesser increment; thus, arriving at the DFT in a sandwiching fashion. This method, which uses both the step-down and step-up methods, would be expected to arrive at the true DFT value. These methods will be further discussed in the next chapter.

Obviously, meticulous method to determine the DFT is valuable for setting the shock therapy at the lowest possible value. Customarily, the shock therapy is programmed at > 10 joules above the DFT. In the past, when monophasic waveform shock was used, the DFT was frequently found at values between 15-20 joules, resulting in programming the shock therapy at or near the maximum value. Thus, if the intention was to program the therapy at maximum energy, the DFT determination can be abbreviated by performing a limited number of testing at a value that was sufficiently lower. Using this approach, two consistent successful defibrillation episodes at a value of < 10 joules below the maximum energy was considered as adequate. For example, for a 30-joule unit, two consecutive successful defibrillation sequences at 20 joules would be a sufficient testing. If 25 joules were necessary for defibrillation, three successes would have been required for the testing.

With the use of biphasic waveform, successful defibrillation could be achieved with significantly lower energy. It would not be unusual to find a DFT below 5 joules. In this instance, the more precise determination of DFT would allow programming of shock energy at significantly lower than the maximum output. The clinical advantage of programming a low energy is several folds. Perhaps the most important reason is to minimize the duration of VF and its associated cardiac and hemodynamic effects. Although the extent of this advantage has not been systematically studied, clinical observation suggests that the patients are less likely to experience full syncope. If the margin of safety can be further minimized to 5 joules, the duration of VF can be accordingly limited. With the newer unit, therapy can be delivered after less than 10 seconds of VF, which is much less likely to result in syncope when compared to a typical event with an older ICD system when the shock was delivered at 20 or 30 seconds.

Defibrillation efficacy is also likely to improve in the future. Optimization in the waveform, such as the pulse duration and degree of energy delivery voltage tilt is found to contribute to further lowering of the DFT. These improvements, combined with the incorporation of a defibrillation electrode within the generator have not only lower the DFT, but also facilitated the simpler transvenous approach without the use of secondary or tertiary defibrillation coils, such as the coronary sinus lead, subcutaneous patch, or subcutaneous array.

- Determination of the "defibrillation threshold" is important to assure adequate margin of safety.
- The two common methods for determining the DFT are the step-down method and the binary method. The step-down method, which is most commonly used, tends to over-estimate the DFT. The binary method is more accurate but requires more inductions.
- In most cases using current ICD models, the DFT is in the range of 5-15 joules.
- Further technological progress will likely offer more efficient defibrillation resulting in lower DFT and, consequently, lower maximum ICD energy delivery requirement and smaller ICD pulse generator.

Cardioversion

Cardioversion therapy is a known method for terminating VT. The notion that VT could be effectively terminated using a much smaller energy has been long identified. This concept is also utilized in the ICD, allowing the clinician to use very low energy levels for VT therapy. The lowest effective energy, also known as the Cardioversion Energy Requirement (CER), can be tested similar to the DFT determination. In such testing, both the efficacy and potential accelerating effect of the cardioversion should be analyzed.

While the key purpose for applying cardioversion instead of defibrillation is to lower the pain inflicted by the shock, it should be noted that only the very low energy (in the order of less than one joule) is typically perceived as significantly less painful by the patient. Thus, if the CER is greater than 5 or 10 joules, there is likely to be minimal gain accomplished in terms of patient's comfort.

The CER is also an imprecise value. Its determination is usually limited by the inability to reproduce the same VT at each step. Furthermore, even if one type of VT could be reproducibly induced, it can not be assumed that the same VT would occur clinically. Thus, low-energy shock for VT therapy is commonly programmed empirically and is "backed up" with a high-energy shock.

- Cardioversion using low energy shock may convert VT. The Cardioversion Energy Requirement (CER) can be tested in a fashion similar to DFT, such that its efficacy and pro-arrhythmic effects can be assessed.
- Low-energy shock may not be any less painful than a high-energy shock.

Pacing Concept and Technology

Pacing in ICD is utilized both as therapy for bradycardia and tachycardia. Monomorphic VT can be terminated with pacing using the underdrive and overdrive method.[118] The overdrive method, being more effective in general, is utilized as a therapy for VT in ICD. The concept of antitachycardia pacing (ATP) is not new and extensive description of it can be found elsewhere. However, it would be important to review the critical concepts for effective ATP. The key is obviously to deliver pacing stimulus to influence the tachycardia such that the pacing stimulus "capture" the window of non-refractoriness (excitable gap) and subsequently render it refractory to spontaneous depolarization and hence, upon cessation of pacing, the tachycardia would not continue. The success in the delivery of such critical pacing stimulus depends on several electrophysiologic parameters (see also Chapter 5).

Of the various factors, one can be readily altered; the degree of pacing stimulus prematurity. This programmable value can be coupled to the VT cycle length and be tailored as to deliver increasingly premature stimuli without risking acceleration of the VT. Thus, various modes of ATP are available. Each mode is known by a specific name in each model of ICD.

Among the various terms used to denote the types of ATP (Figure 3-8), the term "burst" is almost universally applied to ATP whereby the coupling interval between each stimulus is constant. The initial coupling interval is based on a percentage of the VT cycle length. The coupling interval of subsequent "burst" can also be programmed to automatically decrement regardless of the VT cycle length, which is also called "scan" (CPI) or "decremental scanning" (Ventritex). The term "ramp" is also almost universally used for ATP whereby the coupling intervals decrement between the stimuli within each group of pacing. It is also known as "auto-decremental burst" (Ventritex). The first coupling interval of a "ramp" is also based on a percentage of the VT cycle length. The initial coupling intervals of subsequent ramps can also be programmed to be decremental regardless of the VT cycle length, which is also known as "ramp/scan" (CPI), or "auto-decremental burst with decremental scanning" (Ventritex). In Medtronic models, "ramp" pacing in each sequence consists of more pacing stimuli than the previous one.

The various schemes of ATP are designed to deliver a series of paced beat to depolarize the site of VT during the excitable period and render it refractory to subsequent stimulus. One mechanism for rendering the reentry tissue refractory is to cause progressive conduction delay by repeated stimulation. Thus, the goal of ATP is to deliver successive beats to the site of the reentry circuit with sufficient degree of prematurity. However, rapid pacing at very short coupling interval is likely to produce new and possibly faster reentry tachycardia. Therefore, ATP is delivered starting with a relatively long cycle length and carried on with progressively shorter coupling intervals, either with each successive group of pacing ("burst/scan") or within each group of paced beats ("ramps").

There are many forms of antitachycardia pacing but they are based on the same principle of delivering a sufficiently premature beat repetitively as to depolarize the site of reentry during the excitable gap and render it refractory

---

The various modes offer the clinician with several choices. With the "burst" mode, the number of beats can be increased without risking applying short coupling intervals. However, this mode would not provide increasing degree of prematurity as much as the "ramp" mode. Based on the background and knowledge of VT termination, the ramp mode is believed to be the more effective one but also the more risky mode. However, clinical experience (see Chapter 5) does not support such a notion.

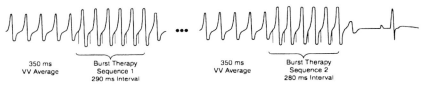

Burst Pacing

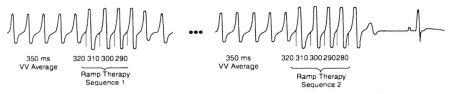

Ramp Pacing

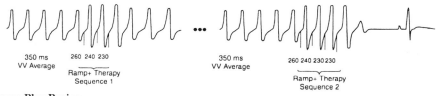

Ramp Plus Pacing

Figure 3-8. An example of "burst" and "ramp" ATP in the Medtronic ICD. The key difference is the coupling intervals within each group of pacing stimuli. The Ramp+ mode offers the option of having the late, additional stimuli applied at the same CL to avoid pacing at very short CI (Reproduced with permission from Medtronic).

- Pacing is useful in an ICD both as bradycardia support and VT therapy, in the form of antitachycardia pacing (ATP).
- To be effective, ATP must be delivered in such a fashion as to enter the excitable gap and render it refractory. This is achieved by delivering a train of pacing stimuli.
- To provide sufficient degree of prematurity, various pacing schemes are available. While there is no uniformity in the use of a specific term for a certain train of pacing, in general the term "burst" refers to a train of pacing with constant coupling intervals while "ramp" refers to one with decreasing coupling intervals.
- While pacing with short coupling interval has a greater chance to be effective, it is also more likely to accelerate the VT.

Sensing Concept and Technology

There are similarities and differences in the basic concepts of sensing in an ICD and those of implantable pacemakers. The sensing mechanism differentiates true cardiac depolarization from most electromagnetic noise and repolarization signal (T-wave), with a particular attention to ventricular fibrillation signals before and after shocks.

Typically the sensing algorithm utilizes a filter that would reject the passage of signals below 10 Hz and above 60 Hz frequencies. The signal would then undergo the basic steps of rectification and amplification. In this case, the ICD differs from pacemaker. To assure satisfactory sensing during VF, which may have variable and significantly smaller depolarization amplitude than the baseline signal[119-121], the ICD sensing system would typically adjust to ensure detection of such small signal. This is achieved by a method that is unique to the manufacturer and is called by specific terms, such as "auto-adjusting sensitivity" (in Medtronic models) or "automatic gain control" or AGC (in CPI and Ventritex models).

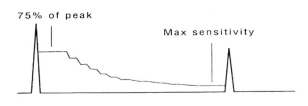

A

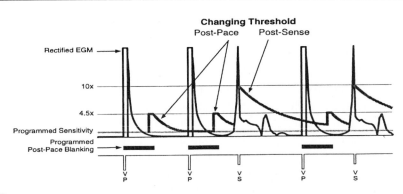

B

Figure 3-9. A diagram of automatic gain control system (A) as in the CPI model, and automatic adjusting sensitivity (B) as in the Medtronic model (Reproduced with permission from Guidant and Medtronic).

Although each mechanism is technically different from another, the process achieves similar goal of increasing the effort to sense small ventricular depolarization activity while still rejecting large repolarization signals. In the auto-adjusting system, the sensitivity threshold is adjusted to a higher value (to be less sensitive) after a sense or pace ventricular signal as to avoid T-wave sensing. Afterwards, the threshold gradually returns to the programmed value, which is usually set at 0.03 mV or 0.06 mV (Figure 3-9). The automatic gain control method, in theory, would change the amplification of incoming signals, also to assure sensing of small ventricular depolarization. In the Ventritex units, AGC is implemented and it can be noted on the EGM as such. The signal would typically be small and at times not detected, but would gradually increase (Figure 3-10).

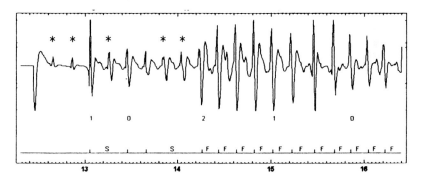

Figure 3-10. Automatic Gain in Ventritex unit, shown as the value below the electrogram. Typically, at the onset of VF, the AGC has to adjust up (in this case from "0" to "1"), but if it encounters a larger signal, it adjusts back down to "0". In this case, this down adjustment resulted in non-sensing of two consecutive R waves. The subsequent auto adjustment to the value of "2", however, corrected undersensing and VF was appropriately detected after only a slight delay.

> **To assure sensing of small and fluctuating electrogram during VF, sensing in ICD is enhanced by a self-adjusting mechanism**

As illustrated in Figure 3-10, any sensitivity adjustment mechanism can still encounter potential problems, especially when there is frequent variations of large and small endocardial electrograms. Such potential problems can only be noted by analyzing the intracardiac electrogram at the time of DFT testing because frequently, there is little correlation between the magnitude of intracardiac signal and surface ECG. Underdetection would typically self correct as long as the intracardiac signal does not fluctuate with every R wave. Thus, if consecutive R waves remain small, the AGC or auto sensitivity adjustment would have sufficient time to adjust. Thus, as shown in Figure 3-11 below, non-detection occurred because the intracardiac signal significantly changed in magnitude resulting in underdetection of two consecutive R waves. However, the third one was detected and VF counter resumed afterwards.

Thus, fortunately, undersensing usually occurs only for a brief period of time that may slightly delay detection but would not result in total under-detection of the arrhythmia. Because such non-sensing of small ventricular depolarization during VF is not uncommon, most ICD models implement a VF detection scheme that would allow for such "drop-outs". For example, the Medtronic units requires only 75% (e.g. 12/16 or 18/24) of "VF counts" to be declared as VF. Thus, a single drop out would not reset the detection window. Similarly, CPI units have a moving VF detection window that would allow occasional drop outs of R wave up to 4/10 counts. Such a window would continue to count 10 ventricular signal intervals and VF requirement would be met as soon as 8/10 intervals satisfy the detection rate cut off. This window would remain to be satisfied unless less than 6/10 intervals meet the programmed detection rate cut off.

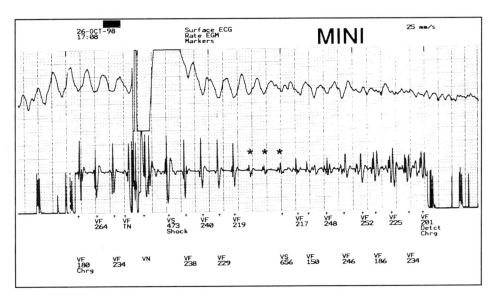

Figure 3-11. An episode of (induced) "fine" VF during a CPI Ventak MINI ICD testing, which failed the first therapy, containing significant signal size drop (asterisks) resulting in non-sensing of two consecutive beats. The third beat was, consequently, sensed as a long cycle (VS) beat. However, subsequent beats re-satisfied the VF window and VF was still re-detected appropriately.

Another aspect of sensing mechanism that is not universal among ICD models is the electrode pair being used for sensing. In some lead models (CPI leads), sensing is performed through the tip electrode and the distal defibrillation coil, known as the "integrated bipolar" system. Some other models (e.g. some Medtronic leads) sensing is through the tip and a distal ring electrode, the so-called "true bipolar" system.

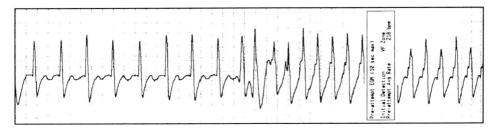

Figure 3-12. EGM from "coil" electrogram, showing VT as a wide complex rhythm, which can be readily distinguished from the baseline sinus rhythm.

With an integrated system, sensing is through a larger electrode surface and is therefore more likely to incorporate far-field signals. Far-field signals can provide offer some advantage, such as its surface-ECG-like characteristics (Figure 3-12). In contrast, the "true" bipolar sensing signal represents local electrical activation and would typically have a narrow electrogram. This can be appreciated in the display of the Vtip-to-Vring EGM of the Medtronic ICD (Figure 3-13). Of note, both "coil" EGM and "true bipolar sensing" EGM can be recorded and displayed simultaneously in many instances (Figure 3-13).

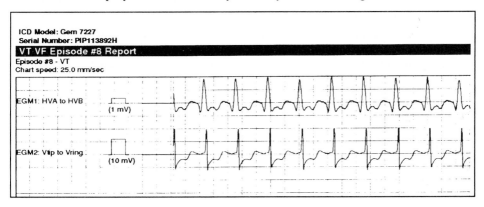

Figure 3-13. Both "true bipolar sensing" EGM (EGM2: Vtip to Vring) and "coil" EGM (EGM1: HVA to HVB) are shown during an episode of a slow VT. Note that EGM2 is typically narrow and, in this case, occurred late into the "QRS" signal, which is typical of a VT originating in the left ventricle.

The "coil" electrogram signals frequently resemble surface ECG to the extend of displaying both P and R waves in addition to being able to demonstrate normal and wide QRS complexes. These features can be helpful in trouble shooting ICD if inappropriate shock for sinus tachycardia or atrial fibrillation is suspected.

> **The two types of sensing, integrated and "true" bipolar, provide different electrograms and each offers certain advantages**

In fact, the advantage of such far field sensing is used in the mechanism for the added feature in the Medtronic units to increase specificity of VT detection. This "EGM width criterion" works through the analysis of 50 sampling of far field R-wave sensing, and identifies a wide-complex signal based on its width and rate of onset and offset. This will be discussed under the section of Enhanced Detection.

Rate and Cycle Length Sensing

The basic method of identifying a tachyarrhythmia is similar in all ICD models. All detection systems are based on cardiac cycle length. Thus, following a sensed depolarization, the subsequent cycle length is measured and checked against the programmed parameter. The measurement of this interval is influenced by several types of refractory periods, during which sensed events are ignored.

These refractory periods are similar to those employed in a pacemaker system. In the case of ICD, prevention of oversensing has even greater significance than in a pacemaker. Ventricular oversensing would lead to false detection of ventricular tachyarrhythmia in addition to resetting and delaying ventricular pacing. Thus, in the ICD, the blanking period after a sensed ventricular event is extremely important to avoid "double counting". Thus, to avoid double sensing of a ventricular complex with conduction delay, a non-programmable blanking period of 100-120 milliseconds after a ventricular sensed event is used. Similarly, the refractory period after a paced ventricular event is also programmed to avoid T-wave oversensing that would also cause false tachyarrhythmia detection.[122,123]

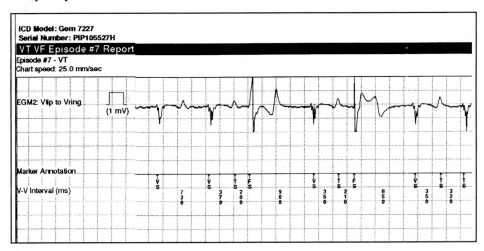

Figure 3-14. This tracing showed an example of T-wave oversensing that was intermittent. Note that the T-wave following the PVC, which appeared larger than those following a normal QRS complex, did not cause oversensing. In this case, T-wave oversensing may be caused by the relatively small R-wave signal (less than 2 mV).

T-wave oversensing can be more problematic than R wave double counting because to overcome it, the refractory period may have to extended to a value that would significantly limit the programming of VT detection rate. For example, if 400 ms would be required for eliminating T-wave oversensing, the shortest VT detection rate would have to be greater than 400 ms (150 bpm). T-wave oversensing can also be problematic because it may not be predictable. A large T-wave signal on the surface ECG or even on the local EGM does not always cause oversensing while a seemingly small T-wave would otherwise do. This problem is illustrated in Figure 3-14.

In addition to the parameters that it has in common with pacemaker, the ICD must also deal with high intensity signals such as cardioversion and shock. Thus it must also incorporate a blanking period after a shock because of the influence of the high intensity shock to the sensing mechanism. The values of basic programmable and non-programmable refractory and blanking periods are listed in Table 3-1.

> **In ICD, blanking and refractory periods are crucial because the consequences of oversensing can be severe**

In the dual-chamber units, additional blanking periods are also incorporated in both the ventricular and atrial channels, to avoid cross talk (Figure 3-15).

Table 3-1. Ventricular Refractory and Blanking Periods

ICD Model	Post V sense (blanking, NP)	Post V pace (refractory, P)	Post A pace (blanking, NP)	Post shock (blanking, NP)
CPI	135 ms	250-480 ms	66 ms	250 ms
Medtronic	120 ms	240-480 ms		200 ms + brady blanking (max 640)
Ventritex		350-500 ms		1000 ms
Biotronik	121 ms	150-400 ms		
ELA	94 ms	172-219 ms	47 ms	

NP = non-programmable, P = programmable

In the ICD with dual-chamber sensing, appropriate blanking and refractory periods have even greater significance than in dual-chamber pacemakers. For instance, atrial oversensing can cause not only inappropriate inhibition and tracking but also in inappropriate assumption of atrial tachyarrhythmia that may result in inhibition of ventricular therapy. In addition, inappropriate tracking that results into rapid ventricular pacing may cause induction of ventricular tachycardia.

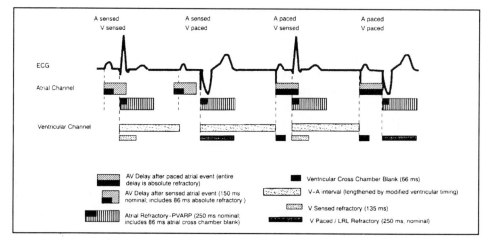

Figure 3-15. Refractory and blanking periods for dual-chamber pacing modes in the CPI AV units (Reproduced with permission from Guidant).

For the above reasons, the blanking periods are usually non-programmable. However, refractory periods are problematic because the clinician must choose a value that is short enough to allow a wide range of tracking yet not too short as to allow rapid ventricular pacing in the patient that is susceptible to VT in the first place.

- Similar to pacemaker technology, sensing in ICD is designed to sense cardiac depolarization and to ignore repolarization and external noise. Thus, blanking and refractory periods are implemented.
- To avoid double sensing, which may cause false detection of tachyarrhythmia, the blanking period is typically set at 90-130 ms (non-programmable).
- The ICD sensing mechanism must also be able to sense small depolarization signal during VF. To accomplish this, a sensing amplification mechanism is employed, known as either the automatic gain control (AGC) or auto-adjusting sensitivity. This is performed differently among the various models.
- Sensing is obtained from either true bipolar electrode or an integrated bipolar system. The latter may be more susceptible to external noise. On the other hand, far-field sensing method can be useful in identifying different electrogram characteristics.

Basic Tachyarrhythmia Detection Features

Detection Zones

In the first and second generation ICDs (e.g. the AID series and the CPI Ventak 1500 and 1600 series), there was only one tachycardia detection zone. Thus, the therapy scheme (which usually consists only of medium and high/maximum energy shocks) had to be applied to VF and all spectrums of VT. Furthermore, it would have been necessary to program this zone with a low rate cut-off to assure detection of all ventricular tachyarrhythmias (Figure 3-16).

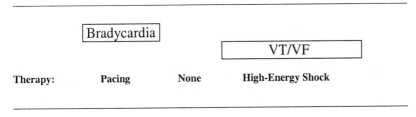

Figure 3-16. A schematic of a single zone and its therapies

In the third and subsequent generations of ICD, the tachyarrhythmia detection window can be programmed to several zones. The purpose of this tier therapy is to allow programming different therapies. Typically, the highest rate zone is programmed to treat VF while the lower zones are for VT that may respond to either ATP or low-energy shock. Each zone is defined by its lower/threshold/cut-off rate.

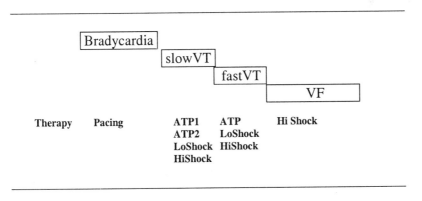

Figure 3-17. A schematic of the three zones and their therapies

In general, there are up to three separate (non-overlapping) tachyarrhythmia zones in the tier-therapy ICDs. Thus, the highest rate zone is reserved for VF, for which only medium- or high-energy shock could be programmed. The other two zones are available for VT and would allow programming of various therapies prior to high-energy shock. If both VT zones are selected, two different schemes of VT therapy can be applied, with longer shock delay in the lower zone.

Thus, in a tier-therapy scheme with more than one tachyarrhythmia zone, the threshold of VF can be programmed more aggressively, at a faster rate or shorter cycle length. The relatively slower tachyarrhythmia, which is more likely to be VT, can be first treated with ATP or lower-energy shock. This is particularly helpful in patients who are on antiarrhythmic drug therapy, which tends to slow the rate of the VT. For those patients with a spectrum of VT, the three zones would provide two VT zones and would allow even more programming options. Thus, for instance, a more extensive ATP scheme can be programmed in the slower VT zone because VT in this zone would typically be well tolerated hemodynamically.

In most current ICD models, the tachyarrhythmia detection is programmable to several zones, providing the option of programming different therapies for slow VT, fast VT, and VF using different degrees of aggressiveness

---

As illustrated in Figure 3-17, programming all three zones are usually performed in patients who have several forms of VT. To cover VT with low rates such as in the 100-120 bpm case some overlap would occur with the range of sinus rates and therefore, detection enhancement features should be activated. These lower zone rates may also encroach upon the upper brady-pacing tracking or sensor rates. In most ICD models, the upper pacing rates can not be programmed to overlap with the tachyarrhythmia detection zone rates. One exception is the ELA ICD, where the two can overlap (Figure 3-18).

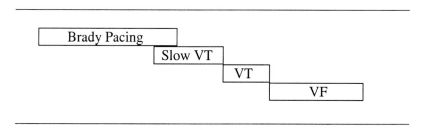

Figure 3-18. A schematic diagram of the zones in the ELA models

Because the patients with slow VT are usually also the ones receiving antiarrhythmic drugs, they would frequently need the support of sensor-driven dual-chamber pacing for chronotropic incompetence. Thus, the availability of such overlap zone may be particularly useful.

In general, there is a broad range of programmable rates (or cycle lengths) in all VF and VT zones, covering rates anywhere between 100 to above 250 bpm (Table 3-2). However, certain restrictions applied with any particular device, and the range may differ depending on whether one, two, or three zones are programmed. Furthermore, the zones are named differently in each model.

In the CPI models, the slow and fast VT zones are named VT-1 and VT, respectively; in the Ventritex models, TachA and TachB, in the Biotronik models VT-1 and VT-2, and in the ELA models slowVT and VT (Table 3-2).

In the Medtronic models, the three zones are designed differently, and the clinician should be familiar with its specific terms and functions. The three zones are named the VT zone, Fast VT (FVT) zone, and VF zone (Figure 3-19).

In this case, the three zones are not exclusive from one another. The FVT zone overlaps with either VT zone ("FVT via VT") or VF zone ("FVT via VF"). Based on their clinical data, some monomorphic VT that would respond to ATP had very short coupling intervals that would overlap with some slower VF (or polymorphic VT). Thus it was believed to be necessary to have an overlapping VT and VF zones to offer the flexibility of programming ATP.

Another advantage is the "merging zone" mode at redetection. When FVT is programmed "via VT", at redetection, the zones would merge and would assure the delivery of the more aggressive therapy after failure of the first therapy.

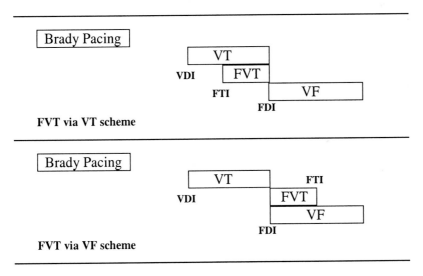

Figure 3- 19. A schematic diagram of the zones in the Medtronic models with the two options, FVT via VT and FVT via VF.

The lower limits of the tachyarrhythmia zones are termed the detection intervals (DI) and expressed in milliseconds (ms): the Fibrillation Detection Interval (FDI) for VF, Tachycardia Detection Interval (TDI) for VT and Fast Tachycardia Detection Interval (FTI). [Note that when FVT is programmed "via VF", the FTI has a shorter coupling interval (faster) than the FDI]. The FDI is programmable between 240-400 ms, The FTI between 200-400 ms, and VDI between 280-600 ms. Similar to the CPI models, the tachycardia zones can not overlap with the bradycardia zone, and the VDI must exceed the longest brady escape interval by 60 ms.

The Medtronic multiple-zone schemes also allow programming of different therapies. Thus, for instance, in the slowest zone, VT, shock therapy can be delayed longer than in the faster zone, FVT and furthermore, more detection enhancement criteria can be applied. In the VF zone, only shock therapy can be programmed. When FVT is programmed "via VT", the three zones function separately, similar to the CPI three-zone scheme. VT that satisfies the FTI would be treated with FVT therapy even though it also falls within the VT zone. When FVT is programmed "via VF", the VT may be treated with either FVT or VF therapy, depending on whether all or not all of the intervals fall within the FVT zone. If any of the intervals falls within the VF zone, VF therapy is applied.

Thus, basically, all ICD models have three zones for ventricular tachyarrhythmia therapy schemes, although these zones may be designated by different names (Table 3-2). The highest zone is always designated as the VF zone. For obvious reasons, it would mandatory to have a "VF" zone, in which only high energy shock therapy can be programmed (although not necessarily at maximum output). This zone is typically programmed at a high rate, such as 180 or 200 beats/minute.

Table 3-2. Nomenclature and Range of Tachy Zones and Maximum Brady Rate

ICD Model	Max Brady Rate (or shortest CL)	Slower VT	Faster VT	VF
CPI (in bpm)	5-10<VT-1/VT	**VT-1** 90-220	**VT** 90-220	**VF** 90-220/250
Medtronic (in ms)	60ms>VT	**VT** 280-600	**Fast VT** 200-400	**VF** 240-400
Ventritex (in ms)	667ms (VVI)	**Tach A** 330-590	**Tach B** 330-550	**Fib** 270-400/430
Biotronik (in ms)	---	**VT-1** 300-600	**VT-2** 300-590	**VF** 250-400
ELA (in ms)	NA (may overlap)	**Slow VT** 250-594	**VT** 250-391	**VF** 250-391

However, the basic concepts are similar among the different models, i.e. the application of varying degree of antitachycardia therapies. Thus, the slowest zone can be programmed more liberally because typically, VT in this zone is expected to be less symptomatic than one in the higher-rate zone. In such a zone, shock therapy can be delayed, and various forms of ATP schemes, such as burst and ramps can be applied first. This zone can also be utilized as a "monitor" zone. This application can sometime be useful when there is a suspicion of a slow tachycardia that may not need to be treated. The "faster" VT zone would usually serve as a zone that is intermediate between a slow VT and VF. Thus, for instance, it can be applied for a faster VT that is expected to cause moderate hemodynamic compromise. This is also an ideal zone to apply the "Shock When Unstable" criterion with the CPI unit. In this zone, a rapid tachyarrhythmia with an unstable R-R interval would be more likely a polymorphic VT rather than AF, thus, the criterion can be applied to accelerate rather than inhibit therapy.

Basic Algorithm for Tachyarrhythmia Diagnosis

In all ICD models, the initial detection criterion is based on the R-R rate or interval (CL). Additional criteria (detection enhancement features) are then applied if they are programmed. These detection enhancement features will be discussed below. In this section, only the basic information from the ventricular channel is considered, which applies to the basic detection method in single-chamber ICD. The rate/CL criteria are then continuously assessed through a moving or sliding "detection window", to assure the presence and persistence of the arrhythmia.

Table 3-3. Basic Algorithm for Tachyarrhythmia Diagnosis

ICD Model		Slower VT	Faster VT	VF
CPI		**VT-1**	**VT**	**VF**
	Count	$\geq$8/10, then $\geq$6/10	same	same
	Duration	1-60 sec	1-30 sec	1-15 sec
Medtronic		**VT**	**Fast VT**	**VF**
	Count	$\geq$8-100	same as VT/VF	12/16-120/160[75%]
		[nom 12]		[nom 18/24]
Ventritex		**Tach A**	**Tach B**	**Fib**
	Count	$\geq$6-100, ave3vs1	$\geq$6-100, ave3vs1	$\geq$8-16, ave3vs1
		[nom 8]	[nom 8]	[nom 12]
Biotronik		**VT-1**	**VT-2**	**VF**
	Count	>12-20	>12-20	X(5-25)/Y(8-32)
ELA		**Slow VT**	**VT**	**VF**
	Count: Y	8-16 [nom 8]	same	same
	Majority: X(%)	63-100 [nom 75]	same	same
	Persistence	4-200 [nom 12]	4-200 [nom 12]	4-20 [nom 6]

[nom N] = nominal value

To satisfy the diagnosis of a tachyarrhythmia, a certain fixed value or mathematical formula is employed. This method is similar in all of the ICD models, but the clinician should be familiar with each model's specific method (Table 3-3). These values may seem confusing at first. The rationale for their use can be appreciated by understanding the specific device operation.

The general principle is to give sufficient time as to allow some arrhythmia to terminate spontaneously yet not delaying the time for delivering therapy because a few seconds are also needed for charging the capacitors. Another general principle is to only require a "percentage" of R-R cycle lengths or heart rate to satisfy detection to avoid rejection of tachyarrhythmia with spontaneous rate variation and to accommodate some undersensing. The device would also come with a nominal setting for convenience, but the clinician should at least be familiar with the purpose and consequences of a particular setting. Basic detection mechanisms of the various models are discussed in the next few paragraphs.

> **Basic tachyarrhythmia detection is based only on satisfying the programmed cycle length and duration; however, the criteria for satisfying these parameters are different among the various models and may also be different for VT and VF zones within the same unit**

In the CPI models, once the Rate criterion is satisfied by both the rate of the tachycardia and the 8/10 count, Duration criterion starts and when at the end of Duration criterion the Rate remains satisfied (6/10 counts) by the scrolling window of 10 beats, therapy would begin. When during the Duration criterion the Rate criterion is no longer satisfied, the Duration is reset to zero and would not restart until the window is satisfied (with 8/10 counts of qualifying rate). In a multizone scheme, detection windows in both or all three zones may be satisfied and Duration is started in all zones. The Duration in the higher zone would take precedence over the lower zones as long as the Rate criterion is satisfied. If the window in the higher zone is no longer satisfied, the Duration of the lower zone would no longer be ignored. The Duration criterion can be programmed as short as 1 second, which is usually preferred for the VF zone, where prompt treatment is usually desired. In the VT zone, however, a longer Duration may be desired, to allow nonsustained VT to terminate spontaneously.

In Medtronic models, detection consists only of satisfying the programmed counts of the number of beats that satisfies the Rate criterion. To delay the diagnosis of a VT or VF, a higher count can be programmed. For VF, a 75% fraction, instead of an absolute value is required, to compensate for under detection of small and variable R-wave amplitudes. The shortest 75% count is 12/16, and the nominal is 18/24. For VT the shortest count is 8 and the nominal is 16. Thus, in the case of VF, the sliding window continues to count the percentage of beats that satisfies the FDI. In the case of VT, a simple total number of beats that satisfies TDI is needed. The counter would be reset by a single beat with an interval that is longer than the TDI but not by a beat that satisfies FDI. The FVT detection criteria work according to the zone it is programmed (via VT or VF). At the end of the count (e.g. 12), the last 8 beats are reviewed. In the FVT via VF scheme, if any of the last 8 beats is in the VF zone, the episode is declared as VF, but if all of them is in the outside the VF zone, it is declared as FVT. In the FVT via VT scheme, if any of the last 8 beats is in the VF or FVT zone, the episode is declared as FVT, but if all were outside the VF or FVT zones, the episode is declared as VT. For an arrhythmia with CL that is fluctuating between the VT and VF zones, both counts are tracked together and when they reach the Combined Number of Intervals to Detect (CNID), an arrhythmia is declared. The CNID formula is equal to VF NID x 7/6 (rounded down) with a nominal setting of 21. Then the last 8 intervals are reviewed. If any falls in the VF zone, the arrhythmia is declared as VF, if none is in the VF zone but one or more are in the FVT zone, it is declared as VFT, and when all are outside the VF/FVT zones, it is declared as VT.

The Ventritex ICD uses a sliding window for all the zones (Fib, TachA, and TachB) and compares the next beat with the average of the last three. If the two values fall in different zones, that next interval would be placed in the faster zone. If either value is slower than all zones, than that next beat is discounted. If both values are slower, than that next beat is classified as sinus and the sinus count. The tachycardia counters will be reset to zero only when the sinus count reaches a programmable number (5 nominal, 3 if "fast", 7 if "slow"). In the case of PVC bigeminal rhythm, therapy would be withheld.

The tier-therapy zones in the Biotronik models are also divided into VF and VT zones. In the VF zone, the diagnostic criteria consist of rate and a programmable X/Y count, again, to compensate for possible variable and small R-wave amplitudes. The VT count criteria is a programmable absolute value, similar to the Medtronic system. One unique criterion in the Biotronik units is the zone-hysteresis window, which allows a downgrade extension when a rhythm changes into a lower zone. This is designed to assure delivery of the high zone therapy even when the tachyarrhythmia is changing into a slower one.

In ELA ICDs, all tachyarrhythmias diagnosis is based on which majority (defined as X% of Y cycles) is satisfied, where both X and Y are programmable (nominal 75% for X and 8 for Y). Thus, the combined count of VF and VT (Tachy) are monitored continuously. In this case, there is a possibility to classify it as sinus (SR) majority or even no majority. Unlike the other models, the ELA ICD automatically incorporate stability and acceleration (onset), and PR association (in the dual-chamber units) into the basic algorithm to reclassify rhythms with Tachy majority (see below). Before applying therapy, the programmable "persistence" (Tachy or VF persistence) criterion must be satisfied. The type of therapy is based on the categorization of the latest CL, to avoid applying inappropriate therapy in a changing rhythm.

Clearly, there are no uniformity in the nomenclature of the tachycardia zones and in the fashion that these zones may overlap. Thus, the clinician must be familiar with each brand's unique terminology and detection schemes in order to take advantage of its features. Prior to gaining full familiarity, it would be best to program the unit using simple algorithm with one or two zones. In such a scheme, there are few choices for therapy schemes but this limited choice is to prevent prolonged episode of VF due to delayed therapy.

- In most cases, the basic detection features are sufficient for the management of VT/VF. However, even the basic detection zone schemes can be confusing. Basically the clinician must determine whether a single therapy for all ventricular tachyarrhythmias would be sufficient or whether separate therapies for "VT" (i.e. ATP or low-energy cardioversion) or "VF" (i.e. high-energy shock) would be more appropriate.
- The nomenclature for the various zones in tier-therapy scheme is, unfortunately, not uniform. In general, there are up to three zones available, a VF zone and two VT zones. The two VT zones allow for different therapy aggressiveness or, in the case of Medtronic ICD, allow for an overlap with the VF zone.
- In some models (ELA), the slowest VT zone can overlap with the bradycardia-pacing zone.

Enhanced Detection Features

Various features for distinguishing VT from other types of arrhythmias have been implemented. In the single chamber ICD, two mechanisms are used to differentiate between VT and non-VT, the characteristics of the R-R intervals and the electrogram criteria. These features are designed only for fine-tuning VT therapy and is therefore only available in the lowest rate zone in a multizone configuration or a tier-therapy device. Furthermore, it is expected that the lowest zone is the zone that is likely to have a rate overlap with sinus tachycardia.

Onset/Acceleration and Stability Criteria

These discriminatory criteria rely on the assumption that reentry VT generally has an abrupt onset/acceleration and has a regular R-R interval. Thus, the common, stable, monomorphic VT from a healed myocardial scar should be able to be distinguished from sinus tachycardia, which usually has a more gradual onset, and atrial fibrillation (AF), which usually has irregular R-R intervals. Obviously these criteria can not be expected to distinguish VT from reentry SVT, such as reentry atrial tachycardia, atrioventricular nodal (AV) reentrant tachycardia (AVNRT), or AV reciprocating tachycardia (AVRT) utilizing an accessory pathway, all of which are likely to have an abrupt onset and regular R-R intervals. Nevertheless, given that the most common situations that need to be distinguished from VT are sinus tachycardia and atrial fibrillation, these simple criteria offer a potentially significant reduction in inappropriate shocks.

The onset and stability criteria are available in most ICDs but their values and incorporation into the detection algorithm may have some differences (Table 3-4). The terminology in the different models differs in terms of their usage of onset and the method it is expressed. Commonly, the change (Δ) from the previous cycle length is used but Medtronic uses the fraction (percentage) of the new cycle length to the preceding one. When Δ is used, it can also be expressed as an absolute measurement in milliseconds or a percentage from the previous cycle length. Similarly stability is also expressed as either an absolute value or a percentage.

Table 3-4. Onset and Stability Programmable Values

ICD Model	Onset	Stability
CPI	Δ 9-50% or 50-250 ms [off]	6-120 ms [8]
Medtronic	72-97% [off]	30-100 ms [off]
Ventritex	Δ 50-500 ms [off]	30-500 ms [50]
Biotronik	Δ 10-90% or 30-500 ms	5-30% or 20-180 ms
ELA	Δ 6-50% [25]	16-125 ms [63]

Δ = delta (difference), [n] = nominal value, ms = milliseconds

Some of these programmable parameters also come with "nominal" values to help the physician with an initial empiric clinical decision. Obviously, the best guide would come from the patient clinical history. However, frequently such a history is not available and the physician would need to choose an empiric value for each of these parameters. The decision can also be based on available literature on the subject. This will be covered in the next chapter.

Onset/Acceleration Criterion

The onset criterion can be programmed as the delta change or as the ratio (or percentage) of the shorter/longer intervals. Most models employ the delta value. In some units it is only programmable in the lowest zone of a tier-therapy configuration, while in others, it is available in both VT zones. The onset criterion is not appropriate for the VF zone for several reasons. One is the urgency for rapid treatment in this zone, hence, no delaying discrimination criterion should be employed. The other reason is to reserve the therapy zone for a VT for which therapy was withheld because of one or more of the discrimination features.

In the CPI models, the onset criterion is available only in the lowest zone of a multizone configuration. It is activated once the detection window is satisfied. It measures the intervals prior to the episode and locates the pair of adjacent intervals with the greatest decrease in CL, and then compares the value to the programmed value.

The onset criterion in the Medtronic models also available only in the VT zone, but it uses four beats for comparison. After eight detected beats, the average of the last four is compared to the first four, and the value assessed against the programmed onset threshold %. Comparison of averages is also used for the onset criterion in the Ventritex models. The difference (sudden onset delta) is then assessed against the programmed onset ("Delta") criterion. Similarly, in the Biotronik devices, the average of four intervals is compared to the average of the previous four intervals and the value assessed against the programmed Onset Delta limit. The averaging method for measuring onset difference has a potential advantage over beat-to-beat analysis. Averaging would eliminate false classification of a single slow beat as an arrhythmia with sudden onset.

In the ELA units, the onset criterion, which is termed "acceleration prematurity", is utilized as the last step of their integrative algorithm. At this step, a single interval is compared to its prior interval and assessed against the programmed acceleration prematurity percentage (see below).

> **The onset criterion is designed to distinguish VT from sinus tachycardia and is a useful feature for patients who have slow VT or those whose exercise sinus rate may exceed the programmed VT zone**

The data on the onset of tachycardia can be obtained in some ICD models, even when the Onset criterion is not activated. The obtained and stored data can then be used for selecting the value for programming. In the CPI models, the onset data is calculated automatically even when it is programmed "Off". In the Medtronic and Ventritex models, the criterion must be programmed to "Passive" or "Monitor", respectively, to collect the data.

Stability Criterion for SVT Discrimination

The stability criterion, which is designed to discriminate against atrial fibrillation, is also a criterion that is available in all ICD units and as is the case with the onset criterion, this therapy delay or inhibitor is only appropriate for assessing slow VT. Hence, it is only available in the VT zone and, in some cases, only in the slower VT zone (CPI units). The measurement of interval stability and its application vary slightly among the different models. In CPI models, the differences between the intervals is always calculated and averaged. At the end of the Duration criterion, the average difference is assessed against the programmed value. In Medtronic units, the Stability Criterion is measured after the third VT beat. If unstable (greater than the programmed value), the beat is declared as a sinus beat and the VT count is reset to zero.

There are two interval stability criteria in Ventritex units. It can be programmed "On" or "On with Sinus Interval History (SIH)". In the "On" mode, it functions as in other ICD models. The second longest and the second shortest interval in a group within a window (programmable between 8-20 intervals), and the value assessed against the programmed parameter. When the stability criterion is programmed with SIH, after the declaration of VT (with the standard stability criterion), the number of sinus intervals or average intervals during detection is examined. The measured sinus interval value is compared to the programmed SIH (programmable between 1-8) and VT is confirmed only if the measured SIH is less than the programmed SIH.

In the Biotronik unit, the stability is measured by comparing the latest interval to the previous three intervals and it is considered stable if all of the differences are less than the programmed value. In the ELA units, stability criterion is the first one employed in the integrative algorithm (see below).

> **Stability criterion is designed to distinguished VT from rapidly conducted atrial fibrillation and is useful for patients who is likely to have rapid ventricular rates during paroxysmal or chronic atrial fibrillation**

Also as in the case of Onset criterion, the stability of an arrhythmia can be measured even if the feature is not activated, for the purposes of data collection. This is automatically performed in CPI and Medtronic units. In the Ventritex units, it must be programmed to "Monitor" mode. In ELA models, it is an integral and the first feature of the algorithm.

Instability Criterion as a Therapy Accelerator

It should be noted that the stability criterion is not potentially useful in distinguishing between monomorphic (stable) VT and atrial fibrillation. It can also be potentially useful in distinguishing between monomorphic (stable) VT from polymorphic (unstable) VT. Thus, this criterion is utilized by the CPI units as a therapy accelerator, rather than an inhibitor. Thus, this feature can be programmed in the faster VT zone ("VT" zone) to facilitate a shock therapy. This form of shock therapy accelerator feature is similar to the "FVT via VF" concept used by Medtronic, whereby a polymorphic VT would likely to have one or more interval that crosses over to the VF zone and would initiate shock therapy. Utilizing this feature as a therapy accelerator in the VT zone, of note, precludes its use as a therapy inhibitor in the VT-1 zone.

Safety Net Features

When the onset and/or stability criteria are programmed, there is always the risk of withholding therapy for VT too long. Clearly, even with optimal programming, some VT could fail to satisfy the criteria. Furthermore, both atrial and ventricular tachycardia can occur simultaneously. For example, VT can develop after the onset of sinus tachycardia and hence would have a gradual "onset". Similarly, a VT can occur during AF with rapid conduction and the R-R interval would be irregular due to capture and fusion beats. Thus, a safety mechanism is needed to avoid completely withholding therapy for VT.

The CPI ICDs is equipped with a Sustained Rate Duration (SRD) feature, which can be activated to assure that therapy is delivered after certain duration of the tachycardia even in the presence of therapy inhibition. Thus, at the end of SRD, a therapy that is initially inhibited by onset and stability criterion would be treated. This feature is programmable between 10 seconds to 60 minutes.

> **A safety feature is available in some models (such as Sustained Rate Duration in Guidant/CPI models) to assure therapy delivery in case of inappropriate therapy inhibition caused by detection enhancement features**

Another safety feature deals with avoiding prolonged antitachycardia attempts. The Guidant/CPI Antitachycardia Pacing Time-Out and the St. Jude Extended High Rate (EHR). It is designed to limit the amount of time that shock therapy is delayed for VT. Thus, a shock therapy would be delivered for VT when the programmed EHR (programmable from 10 seconds to 5 minutes) time is reached, even when the programmed ATP schemes have not been exhausted. For EHR to be operational, the VT must satisfy the (separately programmable) EHR detection interval. Similarly, Once the VT rate criterion is satisfied, shock therapy would be delivered at the programmed EHR time even if the onset or stability criterion inhibits other therapies for VT.

Electrogram Width or Morphology Features

Additional SVT discrimination features utilizes the electrogram (EGM) feature itself. Some of the Medtronic units use the EGM width, which is a simple measurement of the width and slew rate of the electrogram. On the other hand the Ventritex ICD use EGM morphology for the "Morphology Discrimination (MD)" criterion, which is a method of differentiation that relies on the differences in morphology rather than width alone. This feature is available in the Angstrom MD, Contour MD, and Profile MD units.

> **The electrogram width or morphology provides another method of distinguishing VT from SVT and these features may be useful, especially when programmed in conjunction with the other discriminatory criteria**

The EGM width criterion in Medtronic ICD uses the width and the slew rates of the onset and offset of the electrogram. The width threshold (24-152 ms) and slew threshold (18-144 mV/s) can be programmed separately. It should be noted that the EGM width method of differentiation relies only on the width and slew rate of the electrogram and therefore, ideally, these values should be programmed based on data obtained during VT.

An EGM Width Test program is available using the programmer to assist the selection of appropriate values for the threshold. In addition, data can be obtained from the recorded value when the criteria are programmed to the "Passive" mode. Using the "Passive" mode, one can also determine the differences between the EGM features during sinus rhythm as compared to during VT. The EGM width criterion can be utilized in addition to or separate from the onset and stability criteria.

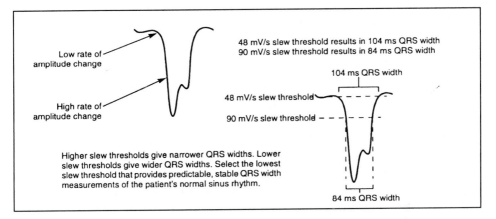

Figure 3-20. The EGM Width criterion. Note that the slew rate influences the "QRS width" measurement (Reproduced with permission from Medtronic).

The EGM morphology criterion in the Ventritex models uses the difference between the EGM morphology during VT to that during baseline (sinus) rhythm as a discriminating feature. This is accomplished by obtaining a template during baseline rhythm against which the morphology during tachyarrhythmia is compared. The morphology characteristics that are compared include the number of peaks, sequence of peaks, peak polarity, amplitude, and width. The morphology score is noted once the first arrhythmia interval is detected, indicating the percent similarity of the complex to the stored template. Thus, the matching percent threshold (programmable from 30-95%), the number of matches, and the morphology window (programmable from 6-20 intervals) must be programmed.

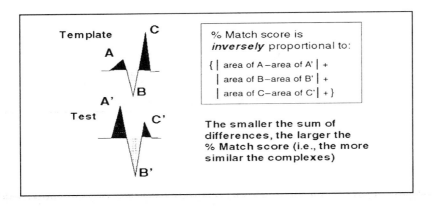

Figure 3-21. A diagram of template comparison used in the Morphology Discrimination criterion (Reproduced with permission from St.Jude)

Data from the manufacturer (Ventritex) indicate that the EGM morphology is useful only when baseline rhythm % template match scores are greater than 80%, when there is no rate-related bundle branch block, and when the VT morphology is sufficiently dissimilar to baseline.

- In the absence of dual-chamber sensing, discrimination between VT and SVT can be accomplished using R-R interval and electrogram characteristics.
- Onset and Stability criteria are based on the assumption that, unlike sinus tachycardia, VT would have sudden change in R-R interval at its onset and unlike atrial fibrillation, it would have stable R-R intervals. These features are available in most ICD models and the values are programmable (Table 3-4).
- In CPI models, a "safety net" is available when programming Onset or Stability. The Sustained Rate Duration (SRD) can be programmed such that therapy will be delivered after a period of time even if Onset and Stability criteria are satisfied.
- The electrogram (EGM) features assess the width (Medtronic) or morphology (St.Jude/Ventritex) of the EGM to determine whether the tachyarrhythmia is wider or has a dissimilar morphology than baseline in order to declare it VT.

Discrimination Using Dual-Chamber Sensing

The current ICD is a unit capable of delivering the full spectrum of therapy for ventricular tachyarrhythmia and also provide a physiologic brady therapy with dual-chamber pacing and sensing with rate modulation and mode-switching features. Such a unit is more versatile not only in its ability to provide various therapies, but also in its sensing capability. The use of dual-chamber sensing provides fine-tuning in tachyarrhythmia discrimination and is expected to improve the ability to screen out SVT without further compromising VT or VF detection.

The incorporation of the electrical information from the atrial channel is done in a specific method in its ICD models, and the integration of the dual-chamber data is usually blended with other discriminatory features specific to that unit. In this case, there is a potential of significant differences in the interpretation of an arrhythmia among the different ICD units.

The CPI Dual-Chamber Algorithm

In CPI units, there are two parameters from the dual-chamber sensing that are incorporated into the discrimination algorithm, the "AFib Rate

Threshold" and the "V Rate > A Rate." These detection enhancement parameters are intended to prevent therapy inhibition from the basic Stability and Onset criteria. The AFib Rate Threshold is used to declare whether or not a tachyarrhythmia with an irregular R-R interval is truly AF and is programmable between atrial rates of 240-400 bpm. Thus, therapy would be inhibited only if both AFib Rate Threshold (exceeded by the atrial rate) and Stability (R-R interval is unstable) criteria are met. The formula used for declaring the atrial rate above the AFib Rate Threshold is similar to the VT detection window method. At the end of Duration, the last 10 atrial beats are examined, and if 6/10 are faster, the rhythm is declared as AF. However, therapy would be withheld only after also declaring that the ventricular rhythm is unstable. If therapy is withheld, the atrial detection window scrolls and AF is diagnosed as long as 4/10 intervals remain faster than the AFib Rate Threshold programmed parameter.

The V Rate > A Rate criterion is also used for confirmation, and if activated, would be used to override Onset or Stability criterion. Thus for example, in the event of a VT developing in the midst of sinus tachycardia, the ventricular rate would exceed the atrial rate, satisfying the V Rate > A Rate criterion and the inhibition by Onset criterion would be overruled.

The Medtronic PR Logic™ Algorithm

In principle, the PR Logic™ algorithm differs from other discrimination methods in its incorporation of atrial and ventricular patterns and their association to each other. It assesses atrial/ventricular pattern, rates, regularity and their association/dissociation. The PR Logic is intended to improve discrimination against atrial fibrillation/flutter, sinus tachycardia, and other supraventricular tachycardias without sacrificing the sensitivity of VT/VF detection. Sensitivity of VT/VF detection is preserved by applying the double tachycardia assessment (see below). Discrimination methods against each of the supraventricular arrhythmias can be activated separately (AFib/AFlutter, Sinus Tach, and Other 1:1 SVTs). If any of these is activated, an SVT Limit parameter must be selected. This parameter is a safety feature, allowing discrimination algorithm to be applied only up to a certain ventricular rate (programmed in CL) beyond which VT therapy would be applied. The SVT Limit parameter is nominally set at the FDI value, such that therapy for VF would not be delayed.

When the R-R interval satisfy the VT or VF Detection window (TDI/FDI), the PR Logic algorithm compares the median R-R intervals of the most recent 12 intervals to the SVT Limit value. If the median R-R interval is shorter than the programmed SVT Limit, VT/VF therapy would be delivered. If the R-R interval is within this limit, the presence of double tachycardia is first analyzed by looking for the presence of atrioventricular dissociation and, in the VT zone, R-R regularity. In the presence of double tachycardia, VT/VF therapy would be delivered; otherwise the SVT discrimination steps would be applied. The PR Logic algorithm would look for the presence of AFib/Flutter, sinus tachycardia, or other SVT, by applying the AF counter and couple code syntax.

VT CL regularity (for the assessment of double tachycardia) is measured by analyzing the most recent 18 R-R intervals and taking the percentage of the sum of the two most common intervals from the total (Figure 3-22).

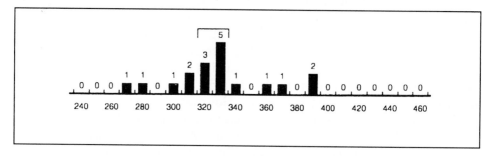

Figure 3-22. An example of Ventricular Cycle Length Regularity calculation showing only 8 of 18 beats (44%) being the predominant cycle length and therefore would not satisfy the criteria for VT (Reproduced with permission from Medtronic).

VT is considered regular if this percentage is > 75%. A-V dissociation is declared when the A-V interval is noted to be changing (the last interval differs from the average of the previous eight intervals by > 40 ms).

The diagnosis of atrial fibrillation is made with mathematical observation that is similar to clinical analysis, i.e. the notation of more atrial events than ventricular events and the presence of very short atrial intervals. The specificity of AF diagnosis is performed through AF Evidence Counter (Figure 3-23), which gives high scores for multiple atrial intervals and low scores for single atrial interval within the ventricular interval. The counter increments by one when two or more atrial events occur within one R-R interval. The counter holds when there is 1:1 conduction and decreases by one when the subsequent event also has 1:1 conduction. The AF Evidence Counter is met when it reaches ≥ 6.

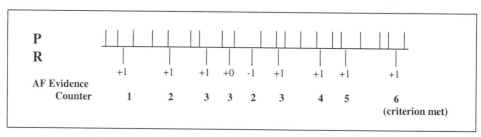

Figure 3-23. A diagram of atrial (P) and ventricular (R) markers in a pattern of atrial fibrillation with the AF Evidence Counter (Reproduced with permission from Medtronic).

In addition to satisfying the AF Evidence counter, the atrial fibrillation rule requires that the A-A median is ≤ 94% of the V-V median and the ventricular cycle length regularity is ≤ 50% (Figure 3-22).

For diagnosing other atrial tachyarrhythmias, where there is a lack of atrial multiplicity, the A-V pattern becomes crucial. The atrial activity is therefore classified as antegrade, retrograde, or junctional, based on the position of its signal within the V-V interval (Figure 3-24). The diagnosis of sinus tachycardia and other SVT is classified according to one of the 19 couple codes. These codes are designed to include the variations of P/R patterns for each type of SVT and would take into account, for example, the presence of PVCs.

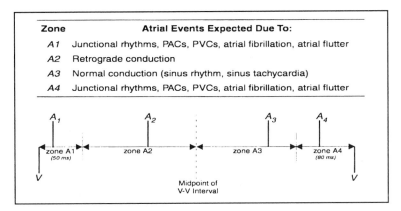

Figure 3-24. The classification of atrial activity based on its location within the V-V interval (Reproduced with permission from Medtronic).

The diagnosis of sinus tachycardia is made when, for each ventricular event there is one atrial event that occurs in the "antegrade" segment (the second half) of the R-R interval (Figure 3-24). In this case, the presence of PVCs would be helpful in increasing the specificity of this criterion, because, unlike a VT with 1:1 V-A conduction where a premature ventricular beat would advance the atrial beat, in sinus rhythm, a premature ventricular beat would not influence the atrial timing (Figure 3-25).

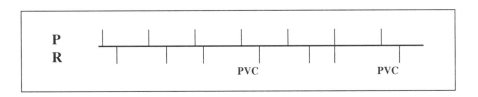

Figure 3-25. A diagram showing the atrial (P) and ventricular (R) markers and pattern for typical sinus tachycardia with normal antegrade conduction.

When 1:1 atrial/ventricular relationship is present, the algorithm classifies the rhythm as either atrial or ventricular in origin based on the assumption that there is no excessive delay in antegrade or retrograde AV nodal conduction. Thus, in a 1:1 tachycardia, when the atrial event falls in the antegrade segment, a sinus or atrial tachycardia is assumed; when the atrial event falls within the retrograde segment, it is considered retrogradely conducted atrial depolarization from a ventricular rhythm. This classification assumes that there is no delayed conduction in the antegrade or retrograde direction.

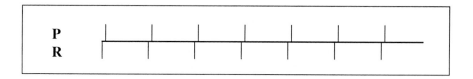

Figure 3-26. A diagram of Other 1:1 SVT, where the atrial (P) and ventricular (R) events are occurring almost simultaneously (the P falling in the junctional segment of the R-R interval).

The "Other 1:1 SVTs Criterion" is designed to discriminate against common SVT such as AVNRT and AVRT. Thus, typical for this criterion is the appearance of 1:1 atrial and ventricular count with the atrial events falling within the "junctional" segment of the ventricular interval (Figure 3-26)

In the case of atrial flutter, where there is atrial multiplicity but with one atrial signal frequently falling within the junctional zone, the algorithm also looks for the possibility of far-field R wave by comparing the AA intervals (Figure 3-27). False atrial flutter from far-field R wave sensing would typically have an alternating short-long AA interval.

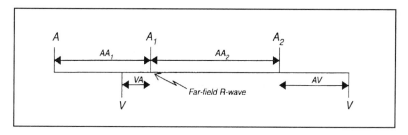

Figure 3-27. Far-field R wave sensing causing false A sensing. The alternating short AA1 and long AA2 interval is typical in such a case, unlike a more regular AA interval in atrial flutter (Reproduced with permission from Medtronic).

When the analysis indicates the presence of both VT and SVT, the Double Tachycardia hierarchy is applied (Figure 3-28) and therapy for VT/VF would be delivered if VT criteria are satisfied (see text). Thus, in fact, the presence of VT is always assessed. Even when SVT algorithm is activated, the presence of VT would always take precedence. If the R-R interval is shorter than the "SVT Limit", VT therapy would be delivered. If not, the presence of double tachycardia is assessed and VT therapy would be delivered if the PR Logic algorithm identifies the presence of VT. Therapy for VT is only withheld when SVT criteria are met and VT is not detected.

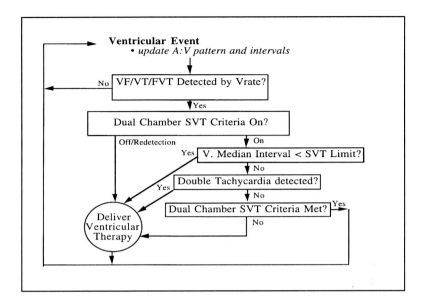

Figure 3-28. Double Tachycardia hierarchy in the PR Logic™ algorithm for cross checking the presence of VT at each step of SVT discrimination (Reproduced with permission from Medtronic).

The St.Jude/Ventritex Dual-Chamber Algorithm

The St.Jude/Ventritex algorithm first analyzes the V and A rates (Figure 3-29) and places the rhythm into one of three categories.

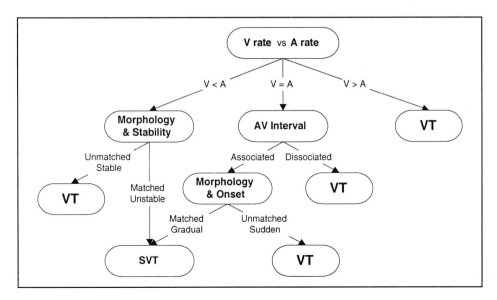

Figure 3-29. St.Jude/Ventritex dual-chamber algorithm that is used in Photon™

When V rate is greater than A rate, the rhythm is classified as VT. Otherwise, other criteria are applied to confirm the diagnosis of SVT. Thus, if V rate is less than A rate, morphology and R-R stability are assessed. SVT (i.e. atrial fibrillation) is confirmed only if the morphology matches and the R-R is unstable, otherwise VT is assumed. In the event that V rate = A rate, sinus tachycardia and other 1:1 SVTs are confirmed using AV relationship, morphology, and onset criteria. If, based on AV interval analysis, AV dissociation is present, the diagnosis is VT. If A and V are associated, then morphology and onset criteria are utilized to confirm sinus tachycardia or other 1:1 SVTs.

Thus, sensitivity is preserved by analyzing the possibility of VT in each step. This algorithm is unique in that it incorporates morphology as a refining criterion. The algorithm is used in the Photon ICD.

The ELA PARAD™ Dual-Chamber Algorithm

Other algorithms offer additional, unique distinguishing features. For example, the PARAD™ algorithm in the ELA ICDs utilizes the combination of P/R relationship and onset to distinguish slow VT from sinus tachycardia. Additionally it assesses the origin of P/R association to discriminate VT from SVT with 1:1 P/R relationship. Thus, a tachyarrhythmia with 1:1 P/R relationship that starts with a premature ventricular beat would be likely to be VT while one that starts with a premature atrial beat would be most likely an atrial tachycardia. Such an analysis would be particularly useful in enhancing the detection of slow VT with long VA interval and in the rejection of atrial tachycardia with long AV delay.

The dual-chamber PARAD algorithm incorporated stability and onset criteria as an integral part. Once the R-R interval satisfies the VT detection criterion (VT X% of Y majority), the algorithm assesses stability and AF would be declared at this first step if the R-R interval is unstable. The second step is the assessment of PR association. A dissociated PR would indicate VT, otherwise the algorithm assesses multiplicity of P/R. Greater than 1:1 P/R indicates atrial flutter. If 1:1 associated P/R is noted, the onset criterion would further differentiate sinus tachycardia versus atrial/ventricular tachycardia. The last assessment, unique to PARAD, is the assessment of tachycardia origin, i.e. the first accelerated beat, whether it is atrial or ventricular (Figure 3-30).

When VT is diagnosed by Stability and PR-dissociation criteria, the algorithm would attempt to confirm this and rule out "pseudo-stable AF" by assessing one additional feature, the presence of a "VT long cycle" (VTLC), which is, in general, more characteristics of AF than VT. This is defined as a cycle longer than the average of the last four cycles included in the VT zone plus a programmable interval, the "long cycle gap". VT therapy is inhibited as long as one VTLC is detected within the last 24 VT cycles. The search for VTCL continues until detection of sinus rhythm majority. Long cycle "persistence extension" is also a programmable parameter, along with other persistence criteria (see Detection Zone section).

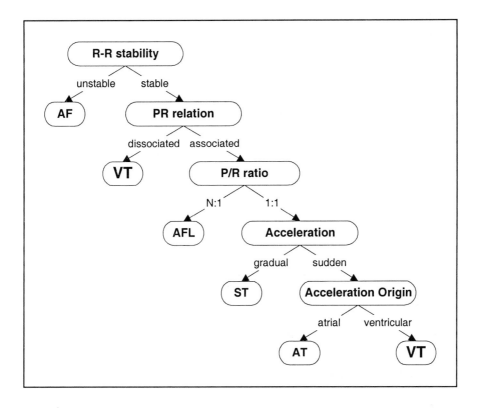

Figure 3-30. The PARAD algorithm. Note the early use of stability criterion and the incorporation of acceleration and acceleration origin criteria.

One other distinct feature in the PARAD algorithm is the first step of the differentiation. The R-R stability is considered to be a very specific feature of VT, and therefore, it is utilized as the initial discriminating feature. Within a certain rate limit, this is likely to be true. Polymorphic VT would be more likely to have a faster overall rate.

The Biotronik SMART™ Dual-Chamber Algorithm

The Biotronik unit uses SMART Detection™ algorithm. This algorithm assesses for many different non-VT arrhythmia types meticulously by but at the same time, checking for the possibility of concurrent VT, even taking into consideration that VT RR interval maybe somewhat unstable. The first screening process compares the ventricular (RR) and atrial (PP) intervals (Figure 3-31).

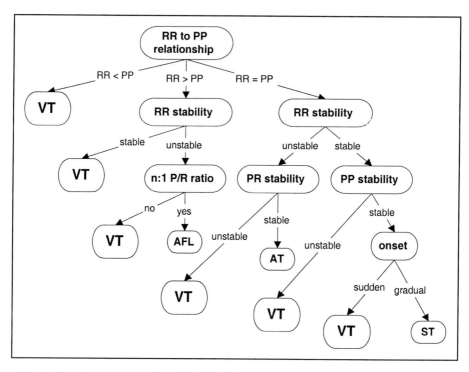

Figure 3-31. The SMART™ algorithm. Note the incorporation of stability and sudden acceleration and the multiple points of cross checking for VT.

In the case of RR < PP, VT would be diagnosed. When RR > PP, then other criteria, such as stability would be assessed. In the case of RR > PP, the atrial rhythm would most likely be atrial fibrillation (AF) or flutter but VT might co-exist. Thus, R-R stability would be important to assess to check for double tachycardia. An unstable RR interval would indicate AF while a stable interval could be either VT or atrial flutter. Hence the ratio of P/R would be helpful because in atrial flutter, a multiplicity would usually be present (in the case of a regular R-R). Thus an n:1 P/R ratio would favor atrial flutter, otherwise VT would be diagnosed. In the case RR = PP, the possibilities include VT with1:1 retrograde conduction, sinus tachycardia, atrial tachycardia (AT) SVT and stability and onset criteria are used to help distinguish VT from SVT, along with PR association. In the case of an unstable R-R, the PR association would be helpful because AT would have a more consistent PR interval than a VT with 1:1 conduction. If R-R is stable, the algorithm relies on sinus interference causing P-P instability during VT, otherwise, the onset would be used to differentiate between VT and SVT. This last step, however, would be helpful in ruling out sinus tachycardia. SVT with sudden onset, such as AV node reentry or AV reciprocating tachycardia would not be distinguished.

The algorithm offers an additional feature for distinguishing the various arrhythmias with 1:1 A/V relationship. A premature ventricular extra stimulus

(PVES) can be used during the arrhythmia, a maneuver that is familiar to the electrophysiologist. In the case of atrial or sinus tachycardia, the PVES would not influence the A-A interval (assuming that its retrograde conduction would be prevented by the antegrade depolariation of the AV node), while in VT with 1:1 retrograde conduction (via the AV node), it would advance the A in a decremental fashion. However, this differentiating method would not distinguish VT an orthodromic SVT using an accessory pathway retrogradely, because the PVES in this reentry arrhythmia would also advance the A. Furthermore, the reliability of advancement with PVES depends on the degree of prematurity. Thus, this feature may have low sensitivity and specificity overall.

> **Detection enhancements using dual-chamber sensing provide more differentiating feature and is potentially more accurate than those using rate and morphology alone, but the clinician must be familiar with the unique feature of each models and their respective advantages and disadvantages**

- SVT can be discriminated from VT using the information from the atrial channel.
- The method of incorporating the dual-chamber information is different among the various models and in many instances, it is combined with Onset and Stability criteria.
- In the Guidant/CPI models, the two parameters "Vrate>Arate" and "AFib Rate Threshold" are used to avoid therapy inhibition by Onset and Stability criteria. Thus, in the event of an irregular tachycardia, therapy would only be inhibited if AFib is confirmed and in the event of slow-onset tachycardia therapy would be inhibited only if V rate is less than A rate.
- The Medtronic PR Logic algorithm assesses the pattern and relationship between the atrial and ventricular electrogram. This algorithm differentiates VT from various types of SVT (AFib/Flutter, sinus tachycardia, and "other 1:1 SVT") while preserving sensitivity using the double tachycardia analysis.
- The St.Jude/Ventritex algorithm first compares the V and A rates. In the case of V<A, morphology and stability are used to differentiate VT from SVT, while when V=A, AV association, morphology, and onset are used.
- In ELA models, the algorithm uses stability, PR relation, P/R ratio, onset and acceleration origin, in that order.
- The Biotronik algorithm first analyzes the RR to PP relationship. When RR>PP, stability and n:1 P/R ratio are used for assessment. When RR =PP, RR stability, PR stability, PP stability and onset criteria are utilized for differentiation.

References

1.   Mirowski M, Mower MM, Staewen WS, *et al.* The development of the transvenous automatic defibrillator. Arch Intern Med, 1972;**129**(5):773-779.

2.   Winkle RA, Bach SM, Jr., Echt DS, *et al.* The automatic implantable defibrillator: local ventricular bipolar sensing to detect ventricular tachycardia and fibrillation. Am J Cardiol, 1983;**52**(3):265-270.

3.   Mirowski M, Reid PR, Winkle RA, *et al.* Mortality in patients with implanted automatic defibrillators. Ann Intern Med, 1983;**98**(5 Pt 1):585-588.

4.   Echt DS, Armstrong K, Schmidt P, *et al.* Clinical experience, complications, and survival in 70 patients with the automatic implantable cardioverter/defibrillator. Circulation, 1985;**71**(2):289-296.

5.   Tacker WA, Jr., Galioto FM, Jr., Giuliani E, *et al.* Energy dosage for human trans-chest electrical ventricular defibrillation. N Engl J Med, 1974;**290**(4):214-215.

6.   Tacker WA, Jr., Morris GC, and Winters WL. Transchest ventricular defibrillation of a subject weighing 102.5 kg (225.9 lb). South Med J, 1975;**68**(6):786-788.

7.   Tacker WA, Jr., Guinn GA, Geddes LA, *et al.* The electrical dose for direct ventricular defibrillation in man. J Thorac Cardiovasc Surg, 1978;**75**(2):224-226.

8.   Tacker WA, Jr., Resnekov L, and Geddes LA. Addressing the issue of dose levels for defibrillation [editorial]. Med Instrum, 1978;**12**(1):10-11.

9.   Geddes LA, Tacker WA, Rosborough JP, *et al.* Electrical dose for ventricular defibrillation of large and small animals using precordial electrodes. J Clin Invest, 1974;**53**(1):310-319.

10.   Gold JH, Schuder JC, and Stoeckle H. Contour graph for relating per cent success in achieving ventricular defibrillation to duration, current, and energy content of shock. Am Heart J, 1979;**98**(2):207-212.

11.   Geddes LA, Tacker WA, Babbs CF, *et al.* Ventricular defibrillating threshold: strength-duration and percent- success curves. Med Biol Eng Comput, 1997;**35**(4):301-305.

12.   Davy JM, Fain ES, Dorian P, *et al.* The relationship between successful defibrillation and delivered energy in open-chest dogs: reappraisal of the "defibrillation threshold" concept. Am Heart J, 1987;**113**(1):77-84.

13.   Zipes DP. Electrophysiological mechanisms involved in ventricular fibrillation. Circulation, 1975;**52**(6 Suppl):III120-130.

14.   Zipes DP, Fischer J, King RM, *et al.* Termination of ventricular fibrillation in dogs by depolarizing a critical amount of myocardium. Am J Cardiol, 1975;**36**(1):37-44.

15.   Witkowski FX, Penkoske PA, and Plonsey R. Mechanism of cardiac defibrillation in open-chest dogs with unipolar DC- coupled simultaneous activation and shock potential recordings. Circulation, 1990;**82**(1):244-260.

16.   Sepulveda NG, Wikswo JP, Jr., and Echt DS. Finite element analysis of cardiac defibrillation current distributions. IEEE Trans Biomed Eng, 1990;**37**(4):354-365.

17.   Min X and Mehra R. Finite element analysis of defibrillation fields in a human torso model for ventricular defibrillation. Prog Biophys Mol Biol, 1998;**69**(2-3):353-386.

18.   Wang Y, Schimpf PH, Haynor DR, *et al.* Analysis of defibrillation efficacy from myocardial voltage gradients with finite element modeling. IEEE Trans Biomed Eng, 1999;**46**(9):1025-1036.

19.   Kamjoo K, Uchida T, Ikeda T, *et al.* Importance of location and timing of electrical stimuli in terminating sustained functional reentry in isolated swine ventricular tissues: evidence in support of a small reentrant circuit. Circulation, 1997;**96**(6):2048-2060.

20.   Roberts DE, Hersh LT, and Scher AM. Influence of cardiac fiber orientation on wavefront voltage, conduction velocity, and tissue resistivity in the dog. Circ Res, 1979;**44**(5):701-712.

21.   Balke CW, Lesh MD, Spear JF, *et al.* Effects of cellular uncoupling on conduction in anisotropic canine ventricular myocardium. Circ Res, 1988;**63**(5):879-892.

22.   Spach MS and Kootsey JM. The nature of electrical propagation in cardiac muscle. Am J Physiol, 1983;**244**(1):H3-22.

23.   Spach MS. The discontinuous nature of electrical propagation in cardiac muscle. Consideration of a quantitative model incorporating the membrane ionic properties and structural complexities. The ALZA distinguished lecture. Ann Biomed Eng, 1983;**11**(3-4):209-261.

24.   Roberts DE and Scher AM. Effect of tissue anisotropy on extracellular potential fields in canine myocardium in situ. Circ Res, 1982;**50**(3):342-351.

25.   Tung L, Sliz N, and Mulligan MR. Influence of electrical axis of stimulation on excitation of cardiac muscle cells. Circ Res, 1991;**69**(3):722-730.

26.   Frazier DW, Krassowska W, Chen PS, *et al.* Extracellular field required for excitation in three-dimensional anisotropic canine myocardium. Circ Res, 1988;**63**(1):147-164.

27.   Chen PS, Shibata N, Dixon EG, *et al.* Activation during ventricular defibrillation in open-chest dogs. Evidence of complete cessation and regeneration of ventricular fibrillation after unsuccessful shocks. J Clin Invest, 1986;**77**(3):810-823.

28.   Chen PS, Feld GK, Mower MM, *et al.* Effects of pacing rate and timing of defibrillation shock on the relation between the defibrillation threshold and the upper limit of vulnerability in open chest dogs. J Am Coll Cardiol, 1991;**18**(6):1555-1563.

29.   Ideker RE, Chen PS, and Zhou XH. Basic mechanisms of defibrillation. J Electrocardiol, 1990;**23**(Suppl):36-38.

30.   Daubert JP, Frazier DW, Wolf PD, *et al.* Response of relatively refractory canine myocardium to monophasic and biphasic shocks. Circulation, 1991;**84**(6):2522-2538.

31.   Kwaku KF and Dillon SM. Shock-induced depolarization of refractory myocardium prevents wave-front propagation in defibrillation. Circ Res, 1996;**79**(5):957-973.

32.   Dillon SM. Synchronized repolarization after defibrillation shocks. A possible component of the defibrillation process demonstrated by optical recordings in rabbit heart. Circulation, 1992;**85**(5):1865-1878.

33.   Swartz JF, Jones JL, Jones RE, *et al.* Conditioning prepulse of biphasic defibrillator waveforms enhances refractoriness to fibrillation wavefronts. Circ Res, 1991;**68**(2):438-449.

34.   Trayanova N and Bray MA. Membrane refractoriness and excitation induced in cardiac fibers by monophasic and biphasic shocks. J Cardiovasc Electrophysiol, 1997;**8**(7):745-757.

35.   Trayanova NA, Aguel F, and Skouibine K. Extension of refractoriness in a model of cardiac defibrillation. Pac Symp Biocomput, 1999:240-251.

36.   Chen PS, Wolf PD, Claydon FJ, *et al.* The potential gradient field created by epicardial defibrillation electrodes in dogs. Circulation, 1986;**74**(3):626-636.

37.   Wharton JM, Wolf PD, Smith WM, *et al.* Cardiac potential and potential gradient fields generated by single, combined, and sequential shocks during ventricular defibrillation. Circulation, 1992;**85**(4):1510-1523.

38.   Tovar O and Tung L. Electroporation of cardiac cell membranes with monophasic or biphasic rectangular pulses. Pacing Clin Electrophysiol, 1991;**14**(11 Pt 2):1887-1892.

39.   Jones JL and Jones RE. Determination of safety factor for defibrillator waveforms in cultured heart cells. Am J Physiol, 1982;**242**(4):H662-670.

40.   Jones JL, Jones RE, and Balasky G. Microlesion formation in myocardial cells by high-intensity electric field stimulation. Am J Physiol, 1987;**253**(2 Pt 2):H480-486.

41.   Walcott GP, Walcott KT, and Ideker RE. Mechanisms of defibrillation. Critical points and the upper limit of vulnerability. J Electrocardiol, 1995;**28**(Suppl):1-6.

42.   Swerdlow CD, Martin DJ, Kass RM, *et al.* The zone of vulnerability to T wave shocks in humans. J Cardiovasc Electrophysiol, 1997;**8**(2):145-154.

43.   Hwang C, Swerdlow CD, Kass RM, *et al.* Upper limit of vulnerability reliably predicts the defibrillation threshold in humans. Circulation, 1994;**90**(5):2308-2314.

44.   Swerdlow CD, Ahern T, Kass RM, *et al.* Upper limit of vulnerability is a good estimator of shock strength associated with 90% probability of successful defibrillation in humans with transvenous implantable cardioverter-defibrillators. J Am Coll Cardiol, 1996;**27**(5):1112-1118.

45.   Swerdlow CD, Davie S, Ahern T, *et al.* Comparative reproducibility of defibrillation threshold and upper limit of vulnerability. Pacing Clin Electrophysiol, 1996;**19**(12 Pt 1):2103-2111.

46.   Chen PS, Swerdlow CD, Hwang C, *et al.* Current concepts of ventricular defibrillation. J Cardiovasc Electrophysiol, 1998;**9**(5):553-562.

47.   Jones DL, Klein GJ, Guiraudon GM, *et al.* Internal cardiac defibrillation in man: pronounced improvement with sequential pulse delivery to two different lead orientations. Circulation, 1986;**73**(3):484-491.

48.   Bourland JD, Tacker WA, Jr., Wessale JL, *et al.* Sequential pulse defibrillation for implantable defibrillators. Med Instrum, 1986;**20**(3):138-142.

49.   Kallok MJ, Bourland JD, Tacker WA, *et al.* Optimization of epicardial electrode size and implant site for reduced sequential pulse defibrillation thresholds. Med Instrum, 1986;**20**(1):36-39.

50.   Jones DL, Klein GJ, Guiraudon GM, *et al.* Sequential pulse defibrillation in man: comparison of thresholds in normal subjects and those with cardiac disease. Med Instrum, 1987;**21**(3):166-169.

51.   Bardy GH, Stewart RB, Ivey TD, *et al.* Intraoperative comparison of sequential-pulse and single-pulse defibrillation in candidates for automatic implantable defibrillators. Am J Cardiol, 1987;**60**(7):618-624.

52.   Bardy GH, Ivey TD, Allen MD, *et al.* Prospective comparison of sequential pulse and single pulse defibrillation with use of two different clinically available systems. J Am Coll Cardiol, 1989;**14**(1):165-171.

53.   Hammel D, Block M, Hachenberg T, *et al.* Implantable cardioverter/defibrillators (ICD): a new lead-system using transvenous-subcutaneous approach in patients with prior cardiac surgery [see comments]. Eur J Cardiothorac Surg, 1991;**5**(6):315-318.

54.   Dixon EG, Tang AS, Wolf PD, *et al.* Improved defibrillation thresholds with large contoured epicardial electrodes and biphasic waveforms. Circulation, 1987;**76**(5):1176-1184.

55.   Winkle RA, Mead RH, Ruder MA, *et al.* Improved low energy defibrillation efficacy in man with the use of a biphasic truncated exponential waveform. Am Heart J, 1989;**117**(1):122-127.

56.   Fain ES, Sweeney MB, and Franz MR. Improved internal defibrillation efficacy with a biphasic waveform. Am Heart J, 1989;**117**(2):358-364.

57.   Bardy GH, Ivey TD, Allen MD, *et al.* A prospective randomized evaluation of biphasic versus monophasic waveform pulses on defibrillation efficacy in humans. J Am Coll Cardiol, 1989;**14**(3):728-733.

58.   Zhou XH, Knisley SB, Wolf PD, *et al.* Prolongation of repolarization time by electric field stimulation with monophasic and biphasic shocks in open-chest dogs. Circ Res, 1991;**68**(6):1761-1767.

59.   Jones JL, Swartz JF, Jones RE, *et al.* Increasing fibrillation duration enhances relative asymmetrical biphasic versus monophasic defibrillator waveform efficacy. Circ Res, 1990;**67**(2):376-384.

60.   Murakawa Y, Yamashita T, Sezaki K, *et al.* Postshock recovery interval of relatively refractory myocardium as a possible explanation for disparate defibrillation efficacy between monophasic and biphasic waveforms. Pacing Clin Electrophysiol, 1998;**21**(6):1247-1253.

61.   Huang J, KenKnight BH, Walcott GP, *et al.* Effects of transvenous electrode polarity and waveform duration on the relationship between defibrillation threshold and upper limit of vulnerability. Circulation, 1997;**96**(4):1351-1359.

62.   Keelan ET, Sra JS, Axtell K, *et al.* The effect of polarity of the initial phase of a biphasic shock waveform on the defibrillation threshold of pectorally implanted defibrillators. Pacing Clin Electrophysiol, 1997;**20**(2 Pt 1):337-342.

63.   Olsovsky MR, Shorofsky SR, and Gold MR. Effect of shock polarity on biphasic defibriliation thresholds using an active pectoral lead system. J Cardiovasc Electrophysiol, 1998;**9**(4):350-354.

64.   Roberts PR, Allen S, Smith DC, *et al.* Improved efficacy of anodal biphasic defibrillation shocks following a failed defibrillation attempt. Pacing Clin Electrophysiol, 1999;**22**(12):1753-1759.

65.   Schauerte P, Stellbrink C, Schondube FA, *et al.* Polarity reversal improves defibrillation efficacy in patients undergoing transvenous cardioverter defibrillator implantation with biphasic shocks. Pacing Clin Electrophysiol, 1997;**20**(2 Pt 1):301-306.

66.   Shorofsky SR and Gold MR. Effects of waveform and polarity on defibrillation thresholds in humans using a transvenous lead system. Am J Cardiol, 1996;**78**(3):313-316.

67.   Natale A, Sra J, Dhala A, *et al.* Effects of initial polarity on defibrillation threshold with biphasic pulses. Pacing Clin Electrophysiol, 1995;**18**(10):1889-1893.

68.   Yamanouchi Y, Mowrey KA, Nadzam GR, *et al.* Effects of polarity on defibrillation thresholds using a biphasic waveform in a hot can electrode system. Pacing Clin Electrophysiol, 1997;**20**(12 Pt 1):2911-2916.

69.   Neuzner J, Pitschner HF, Schwarz T, *et al.* Effects of electrode polarity on defibrillation thresholds in biphasic endocardial defibrillation. Am J Cardiol, 1996;**78**(1):96-97.

70.   Cooper RA, Wallenius ST, Smith WM, *et al.* The effect of phase separation on biphasic waveform defibrillation. Pacing Clin Electrophysiol, 1993;**16**(3 Pt 1):471-482.

71.   Walcott GP, Walker RG, Cates AW, *et al.* Choosing the optimal monophasic and biphasic waveforms for ventricular defibrillation. J Cardiovasc Electrophysiol, 1995;**6**(9):737-750.

72.   Swerdlow CD, Kass RM, Davie S, *et al.* Short biphasic pulses from 90 microfarad capacitors lower defibrillation threshold. Pacing Clin Electrophysiol, 1996;**19**(7):1053-1060.

73.   Schauerte P, Schondube FA, Grossmann M, *et al.* Influence of phase duration of biphasic waveforms on defibrillation energy requirements with a 70-microF capacitance. Circulation, 1998;**97**(20):2073-2078.

74.   Geddes LA, Bourland JD, and Tacker WA. Energy and current requirements for ventricular defibrillation using trapezoidal waves. Am J Physiol, 1980;**238**(2):H231-236.

75.   Wessale JL, Bourland JD, Tacker WA, *et al.* Bipolar catheter defibrillation in dogs using trapezoidal waveforms of various tilts. J Electrocardiol, 1980;**13**(4):359-365.

76.   Hinds M, Ayers GM, Bourland JD, *et al.* Comparison of the efficacy of defibrillation with the damped sine and constant-tilt current waveforms in the intact animal. Med Instrum, 1987;**21**(2):92-96.

77.   Poole JE, Bardy GH, Kudenchuk PJ, *et al.* Prospective randomized comparison of biphasic waveform tilt using a unipolar defibrillation system. Pacing Clin Electrophysiol, 1995;**18**(7):1369-1373.

78. Shorofsky SR, Foster AH, and Gold MR. Effect of waveform tilt on defibrillation thresholds in humans. J Cardiovasc Electrophysiol, 1997;**8**(5):496-501.

79. Block M and Breithardt G. Optimizing defibrillation through improved waveforms. Pacing Clin Electrophysiol, 1995;**18**(3 Pt 2):526-538.

80. Swartz JF, Fletcher RD, and Karasik PE. Optimization of biphasic waveforms for human nonthoracotomy defibrillation. Circulation, 1993;**88**(6):2646-2654.

81. Strickberger SA, Hummel JD, Horwood LE, et al. Effect of shock polarity on ventricular defibrillation threshold using a transvenous lead system. J Am Coll Cardiol, 1994;**24**(4):1069-1072.

82. Devanathan T, Sluetz JE, and Young KA. In vivo thrombogenicity of implantable cardiac pacing leads. Biomater Med Devices Artif Organs, 1980;**8**(4):369-379.

83. Pande GS. Thermoplastic polyurethanes as insulating materials for long-life cardiac pacing leads. Pacing Clin Electrophysiol, 1983;**6**(5 Pt 1):858-867.

84. Bruck SD and Mueller EP. Materials aspects of implantable cardiac pacemaker leads. Med Prog Technol, 1988;**13**(3):149-160.

85. Furman S, Benedek ZM, Andrews CA, et al. Long-term follow-up of pacemaker lead systems: establishment of standards of quality. Pacing Clin Electrophysiol, 1995;**18**(2):271-285.

86. Kertes P, Mond H, Sloman G, et al. Comparison of lead complications with polyurethane tined, silicone rubber tined, and wedge tip leads: clinical experience with 822 ventricular endocardial lads. Pacing Clin Electrophysiol, 1983;**6**(5 Pt 1):957-962.

87. Barbaro V, Bosi C, Caiazza S, et al. Implant effects on polyurethane and silicone cardiac pacing leads in humans: insulation measurements and SEM observations. Biomaterials, 1985;**6**(1):28-32.

88. Sethi KK, Pandit N, Bhargava M, et al. Long term performance of silicone insulated and polyurethane insulated cardiac pacing leads. Indian Heart J, 1992;**44**(3):145-149.

89. de Voogt WG. Pacemaker leads: performance and progress. Am J Cardiol, 1999;**83**(5B):187D-191D.

90. Dolezel B, Adamirova L, Vondracek P, et al. In vivo degradation of polymers. II. Change of mechanical properties and cross-link density in silicone rubber pacemaker lead insulations during long-term implantation in the human body. Biomaterials, 1989;**10**(6):387-392.

91. Antonelli D, Rosenfeld T, Freedberg NA, et al. Insulation lead failure: is it a matter of insulation coating, venous approach, or both? Pacing Clin Electrophysiol, 1998;**21**(2):418-421.

92. Mugica J, Daubert JC, Lazarus B, et al. Is polyurethane lead insulation still controversial? Pacing Clin Electrophysiol, 1992;**15**(11 Pt 2):1967-1970.

93. Tengvall P and Lundstrom I. Physico-chemical considerations of titanium as a biomaterial. Clin Mater, 1992;**9**(2):115-134.

94. Wiegand UK, Zhdanov A, Stammwitz E, et al. Electrophysiological performance of a bipolar membrane-coated titanium nitride electrode: a randomized comparison of steroid and nonsteroid lead designs. Pacing Clin Electrophysiol, 1999;**22**(6 Pt 1):935-941.

95. Bourke JP, Jameson S, Howell L, et al. "Are the differences between 'high performance' pacing leads clinically significant? A comparison of sintered platinum and activated carbon". Int J Artif Organs, 1987;**10**(1):61-65.

96. Bourke JP, Howell L, Murray A, et al. Do electrode and lead design differences for permanent cardiac pacing translate into clinically demonstrable differences? (Comparison of sintered platinum and activated vitreous and porous carbon electrodes). Pacing Clin Electrophysiol, 1989;**12**(8):1419-1425.

97. Karpawich PP, Stokes KB, Helland JR, et al. A new low threshold platinized epicardial pacing electrode: comparative evaluation in immature canines. Pacing Clin Electrophysiol, 1988;**11**(8):1139-1148.

98. Midei MG, Jones BR, and Brinker JA. A comparison of platinized grooved electrode performance with ring-tip electrodes. Pacing Clin Electrophysiol, 1989;**12**(5):752-756.

99. Stewart S, Cohen J, and Murphy G. Sutureless epicardial pacemaker lead: a satisfactory preliminary experience. Chest, 1975;**67**(5):564-567.

100. Stokes K and Bird T. A new efficient NanoTip lead. Pacing Clin Electrophysiol, 1990;**13**(12 Pt 2):1901-1905.

101. Wiegand UK, Potratz J, Luninghake F, et al. Electrophysiological characteristics of bipolar membrane carbon leads with and without steroid elution compared with a conventional carbon and a steroid-eluting platinum lead. Pacing Clin Electrophysiol, 1996;**19**(8):1155-1161.

102. Molajo AO, Bowes RJ, Fananapazir L, et al. Comparison of vitreous carbon and elgiloy transvenous ventricular pacing leads. Pacing Clin Electrophysiol, 1985;**8**(2):261-265.

103. Pioger G and Garberoglio B. Pacemaker electrodes and problems related to cardiac pacing and sensing: current solutions and future trends. Life Support Syst, 1984;**2**(3):169-181.

104.   Jung W, Manz M, Moosdorf R, *et al.* Failure of an implantable cardioverter-defibrillator to redetect ventricular fibrillation in patients with a nonthoracotomy lead system [see comments]. Circulation, 1992;**86**(4):1217-1222.

105.   Greatbatch W and Holmes CF. The lithium/iodine battery: a historical perspective. Pacing Clin Electrophysiol, 1992;**15**(11 Pt 2):2034-2036.

106.   Takeuchi E and Quattrini J. Batteries for implantable defibrillators. Med Electronics, 1989;**119**:114-117.

107.   Swerdlow CD, Kass RM, Chen PS, *et al.* Effect of capacitor size and pathway resistance on defibrillation threshold for implantable defibrillators. Circulation, 1994;**90**(4):1840-1846.

108.   Leonelli FM, Kroll MW, and Brewer JE. Defibrillation thresholds are lower with smaller storage capacitors. Pacing Clin Electrophysiol, 1995;**18**(9 Pt 1):1661-1665.

109.   Alt E, Evans F, Wolf PD, *et al.* Does reducing capacitance have potential for further miniaturisation of implantable defibrillators? Heart, 1997;**77**(3):234-237.

110.   Winkle RA, Mead RH, Ruder MA, *et al.* Effect of duration of ventricular fibrillation on defibrillation efficacy in humans. Circulation, 1990;**81**(5):1477-1481.

111.   Bardy GH, Ivey TD, Allen M, *et al.* A prospective, randomized evaluation of effect of ventricular fibrillation duration on defibrillation thresholds in humans. J Am Coll Cardiol, 1989;**13**(6):1362-1366.

112.   Zhou X, Daubert JP, Wolf PD, *et al.* Epicardial mapping of ventricular defibrillation with monophasic and biphasic shocks in dogs. Circ Res, 1993;**72**(1):145-160.

113.   Bourland JD, Tacker WA, Jr., and Geddes LA. Strength-duration curves for trapezoidal waveforms of various tilts for transchest defibrillation in animals. Med Instrum, 1978;**12**(1):38-41.

114.   Rattes MF, Jones DL, Sharma AD, *et al.* Defibrillation threshold: a simple and quantitative estimate of the ability to defibrillate. Pacing Clin Electrophysiol, 1987;**10**(1 Pt 1):70-77.

115.   McDaniel WC and Schuder JC. The cardiac ventricular defibrillation threshold: inherent limitations in its application and interpretation. Med Instrum, 1987;**21**(3):170-176.

116.   Jones DL, Irish WD, and Klein GJ. Defibrillation efficacy. Comparison of defibrillation threshold versus dose-response curve determination. Circ Res, 1991;**69**(1):45-51.

117.   Church T, Martinson M, Kallok M, *et al.* A model to evaluate alternative methods of defibrillation threshold determination. Pacing Clin Electrophysiol, 1988;**11**(11 Pt 2):2002-2007.

118.   Josephson ME, Horowitz LN, Farshidi A, *et al.* Recurrent sustained ventricular tachycardia. 1. Mechanisms. Circulation, 1978;**57**(3):431-440.

119.   Bardy GH, Ivey TD, Stewart R, *et al.* Failure of the automatic implantable defibrillator to detect ventricular fibrillation. Am J Cardiol, 1986;**58**(11):1107-1108.

120.   Ellenbogen KA, Wood MA, Stambler BS, *et al.* Measurement of ventricular electrogram amplitude during intraoperative induction of ventricular tachyarrhythmias. Am J Cardiol, 1992;**70**(11):1017-1022.

121.   Leitch JW, Yee R, Klein GJ, *et al.* Correlation between the ventricular electrogram amplitude in sinus rhythm and in ventricular fibrillation. Pacing Clin Electrophysiol, 1990;**13**(9):1105-1109.

122.   Singer I, de Borde R, Veltri EP, *et al.* The automatic implantable cardioverter defibrillator: T wave sensing in the newest generation. Pacing Clin Electrophysiol, 1988;**11**(11 Pt 1):1584-1591.

123.   Kelly PA, Mann DE, Damle RS, *et al.* Oversensing during ventricular pacing in patients with a third-generation implantable cardioverter-defibrillator. J Am Coll Cardiol, 1994;**23**(7):1531-1534.

CHAPTER 4

IMPLANTATION PROCEDURE

The Open-Chest Surgical Approach

In its early technological stages, the ICD required large defibrillator patches. In addition, it used relatively large battery and capacitor components that would need to be housed in a large generator package. Thus, the procedure, which was considered as the "gold standard" as recently as in the mid 1990s, consisted of placement of these patches along with rate sensing screw-in leads, via an open-chest approach, either a thoracotomy or median sternotomy. At times, additional endocardial lead(s) are needed. For instance, a "spring-coil" endocardial lead would serve as a substitute or additional defibrillation electrode. An endocardial bipolar lead is also frequently substituted for epicardial sensing leads because the latter are unsatisfactory in terms of their electrophysiologic parameters or could not be positioned due to limited tissue between the patches. These leads were then tunneled to the upper left portion of the abdominal quadrant subcutaneously, where the generator would fit best.

As a consequence, the procedure is associated with a small but not insignificant rate of mortality and frequent pulmonary morbidity, resulting in extended hospitalization. Furthermore, the postoperative pain from a thoracotomy, which is the common approach for ICD surgery, is usually more protracted than from a median sternotomy. There are simpler alternatives to the median sternotomy or anterior thoracotomy exposure, such as the subxyphoid or subcostal access, which would reduce such morbidity. However, with these approaches, optimal exposure is sacrificed and consequently, achievement of optimal DFT may be compromised.

Nowadays, an open-chest surgical approach is rarely performed because the transvenous method is much simpler and carries much less mortality and morbidity. However, the open-chest method remains a viable option and in some cases, provides the only safe method. For example are cases where a transvenous passage of endocardial lead is not possible, such as in patients with vascular anomalies (Figure 4-1); or unsafe, such as in patients with artificial tricuspid valves or single ventricle. However, when there is a choice between an epicardial and endocardial implantation approaches, the transvenous method is preferred. In addition to the fact that it is a simpler to perform, endocardial system also has the potential advantage of having better lead performance and longevity. However, these issues remain speculative because there has not been sufficient follow up of the endocardial lead system. The assumption is based on the history of epicardial pacemaker leads, which were noted to have a relatively short life expectancy compared to endocardial leads. Indeed, the limited data on the survival of epicardial system indicated that its longevity is limited, mainly due to deterioration of its pace/sense components. In our experience with CPI (model K54) and Medtronic (model C4312) epicardial pacing leads in 204 patients, we noted a deterioration rate of 18% at 58 months; compared to 7% of tunneled endocardial leads in 191 patients at 48 months. In our comparative study, we specifically include only patients with abdominal ICD implantation. Another study comparing endocardial lead longevity in abdominal and pectoral ICDs showed that the systems implanted pectorally had better longevity than those implanted abdominally. Unfortunately, in any of such studies mentioned, other factors may play significant role as well, such as the improvement in lead technology and the center's experience.

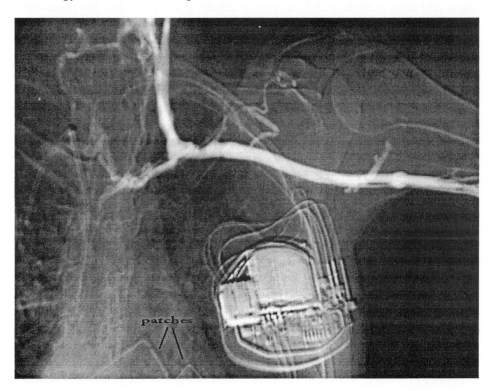

Figure 4-X. An epicardial patch ICD lead system in a patient with an occluded left subclavian vein and a chronic indwelling catheter in the right subclavian vein. The leads were tunneled up for a pectoral generator placement

In spite of its many drawbacks, the open-chest procedure was, for the most part, quite successful and has definitely provided us with basic insight into the technical and clinical aspect of ICD therapy. Clinical experience in dealing with defibrillation parameters was in agreement with the theories and beliefs on the subject. Anecdotal experience seemed to confirm the general notion that defibrillation could be improved or facilitated by the use of large patches, additional defibrillation electrodes (such as the SVC spring endocardial lead), and repositioning of patches. It was also anecdotally noted, as expected, that some anatomical variables such as severe cardiomegaly and cardiac hypertrophy would raise the DFT. Furthermore, it was also noted that there is a certain amount of tolerance to defibrillation testing and that multiple testing attempts could lead to greater difficulty in defibrillating and deterioration in overall hemodynamic status. Finally, it was also apparent that antiarrhythmic drugs, particularly amiodarone, could increase the DFT.[1-5] With amiodarone, it was also observed that fibrillation can be very difficult to induce and sometimes can not be induced at all.

Early experience in ICD implantation provided us with many clinical insights into the complexity of this seemingly simple system

---

From the technical point of view, this early experience provided us with a greater appreciation and respect for the potential complexity of the apparently simple therapy. One example was the difficulty in tailoring the device parameters to the patient arrhythmia or vice versa. Variation in patient's VT rate would frequently pose a problem with the first generation of non-programmable units and the only solution would be to alter the patient's medical therapy. Inappropriate shocks due to atrial fibrillation were another common problem for which there were little options available in terms of programming the ICD unit. Finally, without the availability of device memory, trouble shooting was extremely difficult.

Improvements in Device Hardware

The ICD has come a long way since its inception era. Although at one time considered impossible, cardiac defibrillation with a good DFT can now be achieved with a high success rate using defibrillation coils incorporated onto an endocardial lead system. A variety of coil positions were tested. One coil that is incorporated onto the right ventricular apex lead is commonly used as the cathode. The anodal coil can be positioned within the superior vena cava, either on the same or separate lead, or within the coronary sinus. At its earlier technological stages, such combination of coils/leads might not be sufficient in providing adequate DFT, and additional anodes might be necessary, such as the subcutaneous patch or array system. The combined leads were then tunneled subcutaneously to the abdominally positioned generator. As advancing battery and capacitor technology allowed for smaller generators, a pectoral placement became feasible and, subsequently, the generator itself was used as the anode.

Achievement of low DFT with the non-thoracotomy approach has also improved significantly, mostly through optimization of the delivery of defibrillation energy, such as the use of biphasic waveform. The simultaneous advances in defibrillation delivery, lead, battery, and capacitor technology have produced an effective lead system with a smaller pulse generator (Figure 4-2), allowing for the currently simple pectoral/endocardial ICD implantation. As a result, the procedure at its present stage does not differ much from a permanent pacemaker implantation.

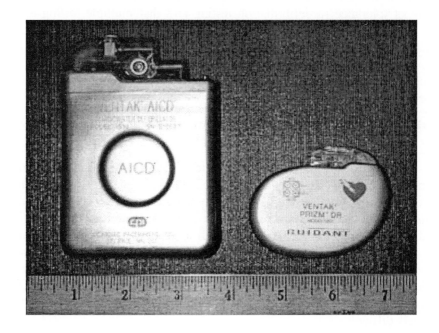

Figure 4-2. Comparison of an early CPI ICD (Ventak 1510) and late CPI Prizm DR

Reduction of ICD generator size was made possible by many factors, such as the use of new, smaller capacitors (Figure 4-3).

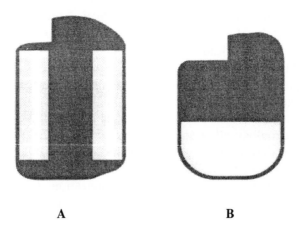

A   B

Figure 4-3. A diagram of older (A) and newer (B) capacitors (white segment), illustrating its impact on the overall shape and size of the pulse generator (Reproduced with permission from Medtronic.

Current Technique

Lead(s) Implantation

Nowadays, the most common approach for ICD implantation is using the transvenous lead with a pectoral generator placement, very similar to the techniques involved in permanent pacemaker implantation. Like pacemaker implantation, venous entry for the lead is selected based on clinical or anatomical situation and operator's preference. The left side is preferred for several reasons. The gentler angle of the left brachiocephalic caval junction as compared to the right, allowed for an easier passage of the lead. In addition, if the generator is being used as one of the defibrillation electrode, a left-sided position is likely to provide a lower DFT.[6] A common choice is the subclavian venous puncture, but cephalic venous cut down[7] and axillary venous puncture are also used. In fact, the latter two approaches are likely to avoid problems with clavicular crush[8] and improve lead longevity. Because the cephalic vein is typically too small to accommodate a large ICD lead, especially when dual-chamber unit is indicated, the axillary vein offers the best approach in terms of avoiding the clavicular-rib window (Figure 4-4). The axillary approach can be easily and systematically performed with the use of contrast radiographic visualization. Accidental puncture of the pleural cavity can be avoided by maintaining a narrow angle of entry to the thoracic cage.

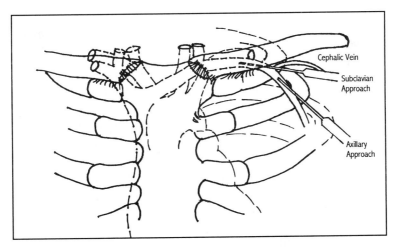

Figure 4-4. The three approaches, cephalic, subclavian, and axillary veins are shown, illustrating how the axillary venous entry avoids the clavicular-rib entrapment.

Passage of the lead(s) is performed in the manner similar to the advancement of pacemaker leads. The RV/defibrillation lead is typically larger than the average pacemaker lead but it requires similar method of placement, even in the case of a vascular anomaly such as a persistent left superior vena cava (Figure 4-5).

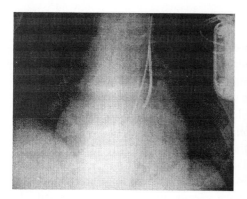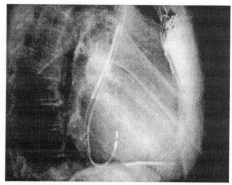

Figure 4-5. Chest radiographs (PA view, left panel and lateral view, right panel) of atrial and ventricular leads of a dual-chamber ICD system in a patient with persistent left superior vena cava. Note the posterior entry of the leads into the low RA region necessitating an acute angle of the RV lead in its entry into the right ventricle.

Transvenous ICD system is similar to a pacemaker system and therefore its implantation should be carried on with the same precautions, including the avoidance of subclavicular crush especially because the ventricular lead is of slightly larger caliber

---

The ICD endocardial lead is designed for right ventricular placement and is equipped with either a passive tine tip or an active screw-in mechanism. The lead electrodes comprised of a bipolar sensing/pacing set and a defibrillation coil system. Mechanically, there are two types of bipolar sensing/pacing lead mechanisms, a "true" and an integrated system. In the true bipolar system, two small electrodes are positioned at the distal tip of the lead and these electrodes are separate from the distal defibrillation coil. In an "integrated" bipolar system, the electrode pair uses the defibrillation coil as its anodal electrode. There are also two general defibrillation electrode configurations, a single-coil and a double-coil system. With the double-coil electrode system, the two coils can be used in a bipolar fashion. However, because current ICD generator can also serve as an active electrode, a double-coil defibrillation system can be used in a "triad" configuration with simultaneous shock delivery scheme. In most cases, however, the single-coil system is sufficient, serving as a "unipolar" configuration with the ICD generator as the anode. In either case, only a single ICD RV lead is implanted for the purpose of defibrillation. However, unlike pacemaker leads, the endocardial defibrillation lead is large, typically in the order of 9 or 10 French in diameter. This relatively large size should be taken into consideration, especially when other leads are present, such as from previously abandoned pacemaker or ICD system or when multiple lead placement is needed, such as for implantation of dual chamber ICD or ICD with biventricular pacing system.

In the case of dual-chamber ICD implantation, a separate atrial lead is implanted in the same fashion as in a dual-chamber pacemaker leads implantation. The same precautions for avoiding cross-chamber sensing (cross talk) also applied. In fact, the avoidance of cross talk is of greater significance. In addition to its usual deleterious effects on the bradycardia pacemaker behavior, cross talk in an ICD can cause significant and potentially lethal effect.

Ventricular oversensing by the atrial channel can cause false atrial tachyarrhythmia sensing and may inhibit therapy for VT. Furthermore, such oversensing may cause erroneous tracking by the ventricular channel and in the typical ICD patient, the rapid ventricular pacing is likely to induce VT, for which, as described above, therapy may be inhibited.

Although rarely observed, atrial oversensing by the ventricular channel can also create serious problems. Such double counting can cause false VT detection, especially at high sinus or atrial rates. Atrial flutter can be interpreted as VT by the device. In such event, ventricular pacing would also be inhibited (Figure 4-6). In the example shown below, the oversensing was also facilitated by the automatic gain control of the sensing mechanism.

As occurs typically, the first cross talk signal would not be sensed because it would occur after a large local signal. Subsequent cross talk signals, if not pre-empted by local signal would have undergone an automatic signal gain, and once this occur, it would initiate VT/VF count and inhibit therapy.

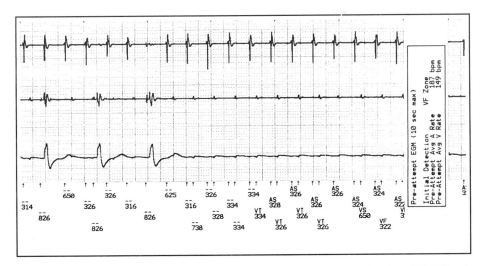

Figure 4-6. A printout of pre-therapy history in a patient with a dual-chamber CPI ICD who experienced an ICD shock following a presyncopal event. (Top channel = atrial EGM, middle channel = ventricular EGM, bottom channel = coil EGM). In this case a crosstalk has caused sensing of atrial flutter by the ventricular channel and resulting in inhibition of ventricular pacing and initiation of therapy for ventricular tachyarrhythmia.

In the example given, the situation was also made worse by the fact that the patient had complete heart block and hence no (intrinsic) ventricular activity occurred, which then promoted continuous automatic gaining of the small signals and, eventually resulted in erroneous VT detection. Such a situation is less likely to occur if a spontaneous ventricular activity is present because the large local signal would "reset" the automatic gain control and prevent an accumulation of short R-R detection.

The possibility of oversensing must be meticulously tested, both during sinus rhythm and pacing of the opposite chambers. Pacing stimulus artifact may have a greater tendency to cause cross talk, but the post-pacing blanking period would typically prevent such sensing. However, the local tissue (either atrial or ventricular) electrogram from pacing may be significantly different from spontaneous events. Such an electrogram may extend beyond the blanking period (Figure 4-7).

Thus, sensitivity setting must take this into consideration. Fortunately, however, such an electrogram frequently falls within the "noise" window, which is the time period immediately following the blanking period. The ICD is usually equipped to prevent detection of such "noise" (Chapter 3, Figure 3-11).

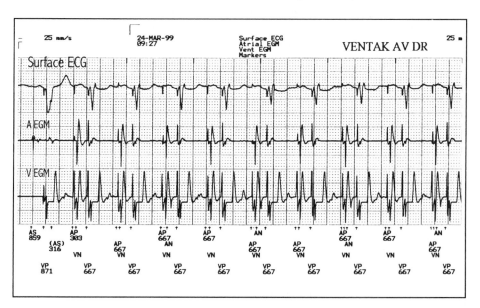

Figure 4-7. An example of cross-chamber sensing (cross talk) events in a patient with a single ventricle and a Ventak AV DR unit that did not result in any adverse clinical outcome because all fell within noise or refractory periods. The first cross-chamber A sense fell within the PVARP, annotated as (AS). Cross-chamber ventricular sensing of the paced atrial signals fell within the noise window, annotated as VN. Some atrial paced events were also sensed both in A and V channels, annotated as AN and VN. Note that the paced A events are much larger than the sensed A event. Note also that, interestingly, large delayed local ventricular depolarizations were neither noted on the surface ECG nor sensed locally.

To lower the likelihood for cross talk, the atrial lead should be positioned away from the tricuspid annulus. This can usually be accomplished by positioning the lead more laterally although in this location another potential negative interaction should be considered. In the case of a dual-coil defibrillator lead, the proximal coil would typically be located across the atrio-caval junction and may be in close proximity to a lateral atrial lead position. In such a case, the atrial electrodes may be subjected to a high energy density during and after a shock. In such a situation, the alternative would be in the anterior location that is sufficiently remote from the tricuspid valve.

In the example shown in Figure 4-7, the atrial lead was already positioned high laterally but oversensing remains a problem because the patient has a congenital anomaly that resulted in severe right atrial dilatation and hence, atrial depolarization was larger than average.

> **Because the consequences of cross-talking in dual-chamber ICD can be quite severe, appropriate sensing must be meticulously tested during implantation of the atrial lead**

Furthermore, if the atrial electrodes are in contact with the coil, there is a possibility of shunting of electrical current during a shock, which may result in suboptimal energy delivery as well as damage to the ICD components. These potential problems are difficult to assess. The best recommendation for the physician is to simply observe the respective locations of the coil and atrial electrodes under fluoroscopy.

- Current method of ICD implantation is similar to pacemaker insertion in terms of its technique. This endocardial method has been made possible by simultaneous technological progress in defibrillation, lead, battery and capacitor.
- A left pectoral placement is preferred as this offers better defibrillation path than a right pectoral generator position.
- Lead(s) vascular insertion can be performed through subclavian, cephalic or axillary cannulation. Common issues (such as clavicular crush) should be considered in selecting the entry site.
- In placing dual lead system, cross talk must be carefully assessed because its consequences can be very significant.

Pacing Parameters Measurement

Once the lead is positioned and secured, sensing and pacing threshold are measured in a fashion similar to pacemaker lead testing. Excellent sensing is very important in an ICD system. An R wave of 5 mV or greater is desired to assure adequate sensing during VF, which can present with a variable R wave signal that is likely to be of a smaller amplitude than during a stable underlying (sinus) rhythm. Achievement of adequate pacing capability is important for the same reasons that it is essential in a pacemaker system; to assure capture at all times and to allow for low output programming, which is key to preserving battery longevity. Achievement of baseline low pacing threshold is also particularly important when ATP is contemplated, because this form of pacing sometimes requires higher output than baseline.

It should also be kept in mind that positioning of the defibrillation lead must satisfy two strategies, optimal pacing and sensing parameters, and optimal defibrillation threshold. For the latter, it is usually recommended to position the lead as far advanced to the RV apex as possible and to avoid high septal or RV outflow locations. Such a recommendation is based on the assumption that the deep RV apical position would provide the best vector for the defibrillation field in terms of left ventricular coverage. However, there is no sufficient data to confirm this general notion.

Testing of an atrial lead parameter is also done in similar fashion as in a pacemaker implantation. In this case, it is important to keep in mind that the atrial channel of a dual-chamber ICD is also an integral part of tachyarrhythmia detection. Furthermore, in dual-chamber with atrial therapies, atrial ATP is a major component. Thus, adequacy of atrial sensing and pacing must be confirmed during implantation.

> **Pacing threshold measurement during ICD implantation is crucial because pacing is used for both brady support and antitachycardia therapy**

Once satisfactory sensing and pacing are confirmed, the lead(s) is secured at its entry site by anchoring it to the opposing tissue using non-absorbable suture. The proximal lead tips are then placed into the generator header and secured using the setscrews. Once the generator is placed inside the pocket, the system is ready to be tested as a fully functional pacemaker and defibrillator unit. Using the device programmer, sensing is again measured and at this time, other factors such as noise and cross-talk can be analyzed. Pacing threshold measurement is also repeated to confirm stability of lead position. Then, lastly but most importantly, defibrillation efficacy should be tested.

Defibrillation Testing

Finally, defibrillation testing is performed. This is the part of the procedure that requires application of internal shocks and makes it significantly different from a permanent pacemaker implantation. For this reason, ICD implantation typically requires an anesthesia team, either for the DFT testing portion only or for the entire procedure. The anesthesia team is an important integral part of the procedure as they provide sedation, analgesia and/or anesthesia, as well as monitor the patient's cardiopulmonary status.

Induction of Ventricular Fibrillation

The DFT testing consists of VF induction, assessment of device's recognition capability, and defibrillation efficacy. Ventricular fibrillation can be induced using several methods. The most common one is the T-wave shock method, where a small shock is delivered at the vulnerable period of cardiac repolarization.[9] It was shown that the strength of the induction shock must be in the range between the upper and lower limits of vulnerability, known as ULV and LLV[10-13], respectively; and the shock must be timed to the upstroke, near the peak of the T wave. VF can also be induced using attenuated high frequency stimulation. Device's recognition of VF can be assessed by analyzing the R wave signal during VF and the device's interpretation of the arrhythmia, which is usually represented in its annotations. The device would then normally charge the capacitor to the programmed energy and deliver the shock.

There are various schemes available for performing VF induction using the T-wave shock method. The differences among these schemes are minor but in some case enough to affect the success of induction. This may be due to the fact that the window of vulnerability is variable and may be quite small in some patients. At its lower energy limit, the vulnerable range on the repolarization portion of the cardiac cycle may be very narrow. This can be further complicated by its tendency to vary and shift depending on the preceding R-R cycle length. The R-R interval during sinus rhythm may vary considerably and hence, proper timing for a shock-on-T after a sinus beat can be difficult to perform. For this reason, it would be advisable to synchronize the shock-on-T delivery after a preset paced rate, such as 400 milliseconds. Such a scheme is now widely adopted by most manufacturers and programmer models. Typically, an 8-beat drive of pacing at 400 milliseconds is performed and a small (approximately 1 joule) shock-on-T is introduced at 300 milliseconds coupling interval following the last paced beat. Figure 4-8 illustrates a typical VF induction.

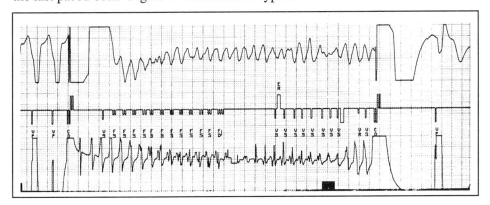

Figure 4-8. A typical VF induction using T-wave shock. Note on the surface ECG (top tracing) that the T-wave shock was introduced at the peak of the T-wave. The vulnerable period extends between the upslope and the peat of the T-wave. In this case, the first few beats of VF was not sensed yet because the auto adjusting sensitivity has not adjusted to the level of the VF signal. Also note that during charging, tachycardia notation changes from FS to VS.

Although those preset nominal parameters would work in the majority of instances, the clinician must be aware of the possible factors that may influence unsuccessful induction. The most common factors are drug or metabolic effects on the QT interval. Thus, typically, the shock-on-T coupling interval must be adjusted up in patients who are treated with K-channel blocking drugs. A more systematic and precise measurement of the T-wave interval can also be performed before hand such that for the shock-on-T wave timing can be precisely programmed. Alternatively, the energy for the shock-on-T can be increased because it is believed that at higher energy level above the LLV, there is a greater window of vulnerability and therefore successful induction would be more likely. However, this assumption is only a generalization of the concept and is not a consistent phenomenon.

If one would like to be more systematic in the approach of T-wave shock induction, the upslope portion of the T-wave can first be measured, such that the coupling interval of the shock would not be delivered at an "empiric" value. Thus, a series of paced beats at 400 ms CL can be performed and the T-wave of the last paced beat is measured.

It should also be noted that the T-wave shock can be delivered in a monophasic or biphasic waveform. Some data indicate that induction using monophasic waveform may be more effective than using biphasic waveform. Thus, if difficulty is encountered in inducing VF, switching from biphasic to monophasic can be considered.

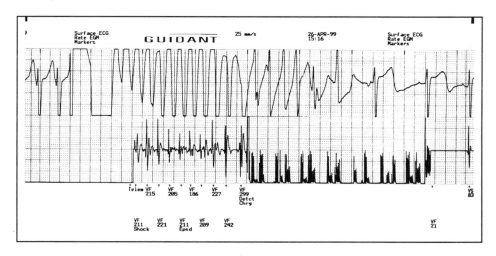

Figure 4-9. Shown in this illustration an unsuccessful shock-on-T induction in a CPI unit. Note here also that during charging, the signal can be overwhelmed by the capacitor action. This noise is more likely in units with a single battery and in a lead system using the integrated bipolar sensing mechanism.

The other common method used for VF induction is the delivery of rapid burst of high energy pacing (Fib High, in CPI models), simulating the method using attenuated AC that was widely performed in the past. With this method, VF would typically be induced after three- to five-second burst of pacing.

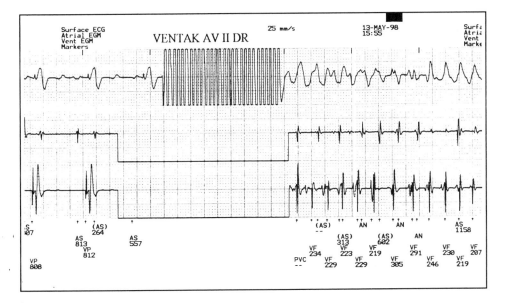

Figure 4-10. This figure represents an induction of VF using the Fib High method (in the CPI unit)

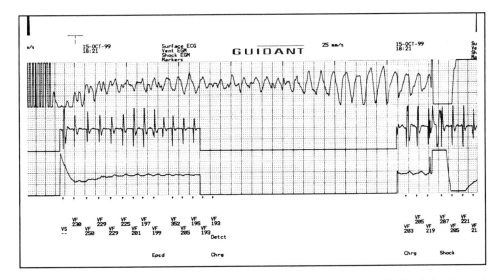

Figure 4-11. This figure illustrates the commonly noted loss of telemetry during induction and during capacitor charging. Telemetry would be immediately resumed at the end of capacitor charging such that the clinician can evaluate whether or not the device was able to re-detect in the event of ineffective shock.

Although it is not as "crude" as the older method of induction using attenuated alternating current, Fib High induction typically causes musculoskeletal stimulation of the chest cavity. During induction, it would not be uncommon to notice the patient involuntarily moves. However, this method maybe more time efficient than T-wave shock because it does not depend on a critically timed stimulus.

The other advantage of this method is that it can be repeated immediately and at any time if it is noted that VF has not been induced yet. It can also be reapplied when only VT, instead of VF, is induced, in an attempt at "degenerating" the rhythm into VF.

It should be noted that telemetry is usually not available during induction and capacitor charging. Thus, one should not be alarmed when the tracing goes "off screen during these periods (Figure 4-11).

Ventricular fibrillation can be induced using various methods; in most circumstances, the T-wave shock method is utilized

---

Measurement of Defibrillation Threshold

There are various schemes for estimating the DFT. Analogous to the measurement of pacing capture threshold, defibrillation can be performed repeatedly with varying the energy. Thus, the "DFT" can be approximated using a step-down or a step-up method or both (the binary method). In any case, the goal is to determine or estimate the lowest energy value needed for defibrillation. For the sake of providing the greatest protection against VF, this value should be significantly lower than the maximum output of the ICD. This difference is known as "the margin of safety" and, in general, should be at least in the order of 10 joules or more. Thus, in most cases using ICDs with 30-35 joule capacity, the DFT should be in the order of 20-25 joules.

The step down technique is the most utilized method. With the goal of achieving a good margin of safety as mentioned above, it would be most logical to start with a shock energy of, at the most, 10 joules below the device maximum output and ideally, this procedure is repeated with stepwise decrease in energy level. The energy increments are, obviously arbitrary but a 5-joule increment is usually used between 10-20 joule shocks and a 2-joule or 3-joule increment below 10-joule shocks. If the first chosen energy value is successful but the first incremented value fails, defibrillation testing should be repeated with the first value. If failure is encountered even with the first value, testing must be, obviously, performed at higher energy. If such setting provides less than 10-joule margin of safety, it is desirable to show three successful defibrillation attempts at that level.

Given the above scenario, and if the physician is only concerned with achieving adequate margin of safety (rather than the estimation of DFT), a simplified technique of testing can be performed. Defibrillation attempts can be limited to as few as two as long as both are successful at an energy level that would give an adequate margin of safety such as 15, 20, or 25 joules, depending on the maximum output of the unit. This form of simplified testing, however, does not provide us with the estimation of DFT. Hence, it would necessitate programming the first shock therapy for VF at or near the maximum output of the device as to provide the margin of safety. If a more meticulous testing were performed, it would not be unusual to find a DFT of much lower than 10 joules. Consequently, the first shock therapy can be programmed much lower than the maximum output, which is potentially beneficial to the patient particularly because a lower energy shock would require less time for capacitor charging.

The step-up method is more difficult to perform, because the first few attempts would likely be unsuccessful and result in multiple episodes of prolonged VF. For that reason, this method, which would tend to underestimate the DFT, is rarely employed.

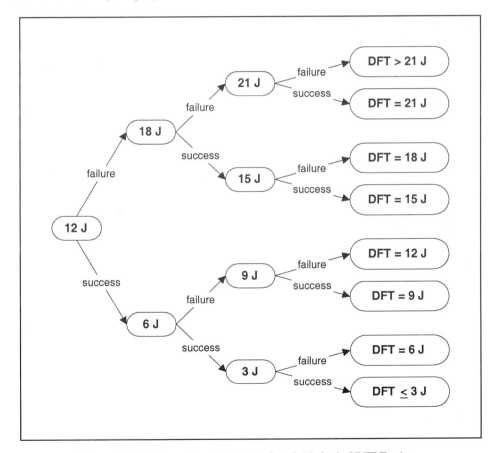

Figure 4-12. An Example of the Binary Search Method of DFT Testing

In the binary method, the first defibrillation testing is performed at a mid range energy level. Subsequent attempts are then performed with either higher or lower energy depending on the outcome of each previous ones (Figure 4-12). In principle, this method differs from either the step down or step up technique because it attempts to arrive at the estimated DFT from both its upper and lower boundaries. This method is likely to estimate the true DFT, because it eliminates the biases that are involved with the other two methods. For that reason, this method is recommended. Typically, however, this method of DFT measurement takes longer to perform. Furthermore, there has been no systematic study assessing the true or incremental benefit of this method.

With either method, a rescue shock must be prepared in the event of failure of the programmed test shock. Usually, this is set up to be delivered by the ICD as well, thereby simulating a potential real clinical event of a failed first shock. In such a setting the ICD rescue shock is usually programmed at the maximum output as to minimize prolonged episode of VF. Subsequent rescue shocks are probably best set up using an external defibrillator. Alternatively, the physician may elect to deliver the first rescue shock from the external defibrillator. Whichever is the case, it should be planned ahead and well communicated to all the personnel involved such that no shock would be delivered inadvertently. Such an inadvertent extra shock is not only unnecessary, but it is also likely to cause re-induction of VF.

When multiple defibrillation attempts are performed, it is recommended to wait several minutes between induction attempts to allow for hemodynamic recovery. If overall cardiopulmonary status deteriorates or fails to recover, which can be best determined by communication between the surgical and anesthesia teams; DFT testing might have to be limited to only one or two trials. In the rare circumstances (occurring in less than 1% of cases), where the DFT exceeds the maximum ICD shock energy, the procedure is terminated and consideration is made for an alternative approach, such as a thoracotomy procedure.

Considering the potential harmful effects with multiple induction of VF, an alternative DFT estimation can be performed. It is known that the DFT value is closely related to the upper limit of vulnerability (ULV). Because the ULV can be determined without inducing VF, this method for estimating DFT is sometimes preferred. The ULV can be determined by performing multiple T-wave shock delivery on the vulnerable window (the upslope of the T-wave) starting with a mid range energy level. Subsequent T-wave shock is then delivered at decreasing energy until VF is induced. With this method, it would not be necessary to induce VF repeatedly and therefore it is potentially a safer technique. Interestingly, this method is rarely utilized in clinical practice.

> **The defibrillation threshold could be estimated using one of various methods, the step down, binary, or upper-limit of vulnerability method, each of which has its own advantages and disadvantages**

Testing of Ventricular Tachycardia Therapy

In the interest of time and patient's safety, testing during ICD implantation is usually limited to obtaining the most critical data. Thus, DFT measurement would take precedent over other tachyarrhythmia therapy testing. Furthermore, it is normally assumed that VT therapy can be programmed empirically or based on preoperative EPS data. However, there are scenarios where VT therapy would deserve some form of testing. Some VT therapies, such as aggressive pacing modes and low-energy shock may cause rhythm degeneration into VF. Hence, if such forms of therapy are contemplated, it may advisable to test their safety. Obviously, such testing can be performed later during subsequent ICD testing such as at the time prior to discharging the patient from the hospital or at subsequent chronic ICD testing. On the other hand, the operative setting may provide the greatest degree of safety and comfort for the patient to perform such testing.

If time and hemodynamic stability permit, it would be advisable to test VT therapy (especially low-energy cardioversion) mainly to assess its safety, because such therapy is known to cause acceleration of VT

It is also not uncommon to encounter VT when attempting to induce VF and frequently, the VT rate would fall below the VF rate threshold. Hence in the patient who is known to have a history of VT, it would be advisable to program the ICD such that VT would be appropriately detected and treated.

Cross Testing with Pacemaker

In a patient with a separate pacemaker unit, special attention must be given in assessing potential negative interaction. This is discussed later (see Section 5). With the advent of new tools for explantation of chronic pacemaker and ICD leads (see below), it may be worth considering revising the device system in such a patient and place an ICD with full pacemaker capabilities. The integrated new unit would be less likely to encounter negative interaction problems.

Final Evaluation

Meticulous evaluation of final lead, device and parameter status is important at the end of the procedure. It is not uncommon to encounter lead migration, retraction or even injury after completion of a rigorous pacing and defibrillation testing. Thus, prior to skin closure, it would be advisable to inspect the anatomical location and configuration of all the implanted leads. It is also important to keep in mind that the ICD had been activated at this point and to remember to deactivate the device if electrocautery is to be used. Once the surgery is complete, the device should be interrogated to assure that the desired and appropriate parameters are permanently programmed. It is also important to provide the programmed parameters in the patient's records such that they can be communicated to the physician and nursing staff who will care for the patient post-operatively. The patient is then recovered from anesthesia and monitored for potential post-procedural complications.

- Measurement and testing of ICD lead sensing and pacing parameter are carried on in the same manner as during pacemaker implantation. Obtaining a large R-wave signal is crucial because during VF its amplitude typically becomes much smaller.
- Defibrillation threshold testing is an important component of ICD implantation. It consists of VF induction and measurement of DFT.
- VF induction is performed using T-wave shock or high-frequency burst pacing (Fib High) method. T-wave shock should be applied at the upslope and near the peak of the T-wave.
- DFT testing is performed using the step down or the binary method. The DFT should be at the most 10 joules below the maximum shock energy capacity of the ICD.
- Testing of cardioversion energy requirement and efficacy of ATP is optional.
- If a separate pacemaker unit is present, cross testing with the pacemaker isessential.

Explantation and Revision Procedures

The need for device and lead revision is increasing. Epicardial leads that were implanted in the 1980s are likely to have reached their longevity at this time. Even some endocardial leads are being replaced for various reasons. Recent data indicate that endocardial leads that were implanted with an abdominal generator are more likely to malfunction when compared to those implanted with pectoral generator. A significant number of endocardial leads in the early phases of the development were implanted with an abdominal generator and a large number of such a system may have to be revised to a pectoral system.

In general, a revision of ICD lead system would require removal of any nonfunctional lead. The obvious reason for removing the old lead is to allow for easier passage for the new lead and to lower the risk for venous obstruction. Another important but less appreciated reason is the avoidance of potential sensing interaction. Abandoned lead(s) can potentially cause noise artifact and generate oversensing that can then lead to inappropriate shocks.

Another group of patients who may require lead removal are those with pre-existing pacemaker system requiring ICD implantation. To avoid potential problems discussed above, these patients should undergo explantation of their pacemaker generator and leads and receive an entirely new ICD system with full pacing capabilities. In principle, this is easier to achieve because the newer ICD generation is now equipped with complete pacing features, including rate response mode, mode switching, and soon, antitachycardia for atrial arrhythmia.

Technically, removal of chronic lead may pose problems and risks. Up until a few years ago, the main method for removing lead is manual traction. Using transvenous approach, traction method can be applied directly through the lead or indirectly using various snaring apparatus. In the rare occasion where both transvenous methods fail, direct traction can be performed through an atrial window.

Direct Traction Method

Direct traction is the preferred method because it can be performed through the subclavian and SVC approach, the operator can have control over the lead directly, and no other vascular access would be necessary. The most effective manner to apply direct traction is through the use of a locking styllete. The idea is to apply the traction from the farthest point into the lead, otherwise the traction pressure would cause the lead body and materials to breakdown. There are now various types of locking styllete available, all having the same principle, to gain a deep access and to lock itself securely but not permanently. The locking mechanism is performed through intertwining itself with the inner coil of the pacemaker or ICD lead. There are two models manufactured by Cook Inc., both are composed of a stiff body and a locking mechanism at the tip, either a loose string or an angulated short shaft. There is a newer model manufactured by Spectranetics, which is composed of a stiff body covered with a soft, fine netting material that expands to lock itself along the entire inner coil of the lead.

In addition to the locking styllete, a countertraction method should also be used. Countertraction is applied using a sheath over the lead body such that a forward pressure can be applied at the tissue surrounding the lead tip. In this manner, the heart wall is stabilized and traction can be applied on the lead tip more safely, avoiding avulsion. The countertraction sheath is also very helpful in releasing the lead from areas of fibrosis along its shaft. In fact, these areas of fibrous sheath are frequently the main reason for difficulty in removing chronic leads. Without the countertraction sheath, the locking styllete alone would not be sufficient for successful removal of such leads in the majority of cases.

The countertraction sheath must therefore be advanced all the way to the tip of the lead. This procedure may require significant effort because it must overcome binding of fibrous sheath that is sometimes difficult to break. To assist in such an attempt, various mechanisms have been utilized. Up until recently, all of them consist merely of variations of sheath strengths, shapes and tip orientation. Various flexible plastic materials as well as metallic compounds have been used with good success. Recently, a cutting sheath system using laser excimer (Spectranetics Inc.) was tested.[14] With this system, the lead is released from areas of fibrous binding by advancing the cutting laser sheath, which obviates the need for applying mechanical force. Early clinical data so far have indicated that the method has simplified the countertraction effort significantly.

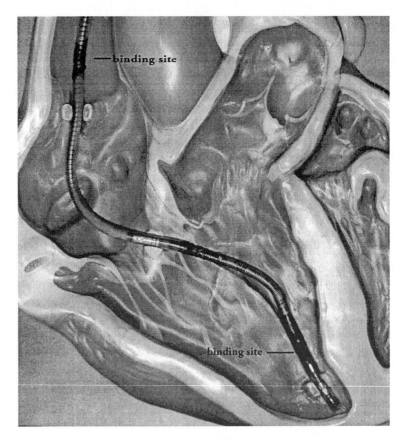

Figure 4-13. An explanted ICD lead superimposed on a heart model. The common binding sites are shown (at the SVC and near the lead tip).

It may be worth to note that there are certain portions within the endovascular structure where tissue binding frequently occurs. The most common site of binding is within the superior vena cava near the right atrial entry. Other common binding sites include the brachiocephalic area and the portion near the tip of the lead. Focusing at the area in the superior vena cava is of clinical importance because this is typically the portion where the laser cylinder must make the sharpest curve. If some difficulty is encountered in this area, it would not be uncommon for the operator to use more force, which in turn may result in injury to the vascular wall. One of the advantages in using the laser cutting sheath is the fact that the operator would not need to exert force, which would potentially reduce the risk of such injury.

Indirect Traction method

The indirect method using secondary traction tools such as snares can be performed through any vascular access. In this respect, the femoral approach offers the most direct route to the right ventricle. The lead must first be released from its superior vascular position. The snare can then be used to trap the lead body near its entry through the tricuspid valve and to apply traction to release the lead tip from its fixation point in the right ventricle. Countertraction can also be applied, using a large sheath that would accommodate both the snare and the lead body together. In the absence of a locking styllete, removal of the entire lead depends on the integrity of the lead body during traction with the snare. Overall, this method is less desirable than the direct traction method. However, in some cases where direct traction results in incomplete removal of the lead, snaring through the femoral venous approach is the only option for retrieval of the remnant. In recent experience with the use of laser-assisted method, it is rare to encounter lead breakage and incomplete removal. The laser cutting sheath can, in most instances, be advanced over the entire length of the lead with much less difficulty than the older method using mechanical force.

Results of Non-Thoracotomy Lead Explantation

The success of chronic lead removal obviously depends on several factors. The national database of lead extraction that registered intravascular extraction of 1441 leads in 856 patients using the standard method without laser showed 86% complete success rate, 8% partial success rate, and 6% failure. The variables that influenced the success rate included shorter implant duration, physician experience, active fixation, and atrial placement. Serious complication leading to patient death were due to hemopericardium (0.2%), hemothorax (0.1%), and pulmonary embolism (0.2%). The multi center comparison study on laser-assisted and non-laser pacemaker lead extraction a higher complete success rate of 94% in the laser group versus 65% in the non-laser group (p = 0.001), shorter procedure time and a high crossover rate from the conventional method.[15] Data on laser-assisted ICD lead extraction are still limited but appear to be favorable also. In our institution, laser-assisted extraction (which was performed after a failed conventional approach) was successful only in 11/14 (79%) ICD leads, compared to 25/25 (100%) pacemaker leads. All three failed ICD leads were due to complete break in the lead insulation and electrode coils and two of them (Guidant/CPI Endotak) were from one patient.

> To replace, revise, or upgrade an ID system, lead explantation is sometimes necessary and nowadays, such procedure can be accomplished with greater success rate using laser-assisted direct traction method

In spite of these improvements in chronic lead removal, the procedure is considered still as potentially carrying a high risk, including vascular and cardiac perforation, which could result in severe hemorrhage and death. Thus, the patient undergoing this procedure must be prepared for possible emergency thoracotomy and cardiopulmonary bypass.

Nevertheless, in the hope of minimizing the risk of venous obstruction and thromboembolism, and to gain more option for the new implantation approach and choice of device, it is now generally recommended that patients undergo explantation of old, unsuitable leads. In our experience with over 100 patients, there has been only one patient who later required thoracotomy for removal of lead remnant from an unsuccessful transvenous approach.

Upgrading to Dual-Chamber System

It can certainly be expected that many patients would require an upgrade from a single-chamber ICD to a dual-chamber unit. The patient with an ICD is commonly an elderly person with a significant underlying cardiovascular disorder who may therefore be prone to develop sinus node dysfunction or atrioventricular block. Furthermore, the management of the overall scope of arrhythmia may frequently require the addition of antiarrhythmic drug. Hence, indication for bradycardia support frequently develops in such a patient.

With the availability of dual-chamber ICD units, it would be most logical to upgrade to such a unit. However, such an upgrade may not always be a trivial procedure. In many instances, the old ICD system is an abdominal implantation. Thus, the added atrial lead must be "extended" to the abdominal pocket. In some occasion, venous obstruction precludes the addition of another lead. Hence, in some situation, the clinician may choose to implant a separate dual-chamber pacemaker.

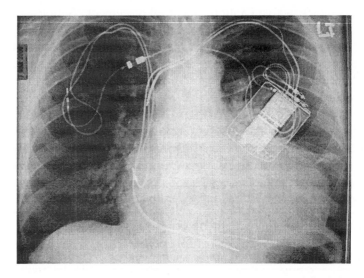

Figure 4-14. A chest radiogram showing a pre-existing atrial lead from a separate dual-chamber pacemaker was extended to the ICD site by tunneling across. This integration was necessary because of negative ICD-pacemaker interaction was noted during a prolonged VF episode.

Yet another situation is the need to revise a two-unit system to a single one. Negative pacemaker-ICD interaction (see Chapter 5) may require the integration of the two units into one. Integration would also be necessary if the ICD is to be used for ventricular and atrial therapy. Such integration would frequently require "relocation" of the atrial lead from the pacemaker site to the ICD site and the two sites are normally located at opposite sides of the chest. If the decision is to add a new atrial lead, the old lead must first be removed to avoid the presence of redundant leads. The alternative is the "extend" the atrial lead from one side of the chest to the other and tunneling it across (Figure 4-14).

To perform this procedure, it would be necessary to use a lead extender but the overall process can usually be accomplished without great difficulty. A special "tunneler" may be necessary. The typical apparatus that is available for tunneling ICD leads would usually be too large.

- Due to its relatively large size, revision of an ICD lead commonly requires removal of the old, chronic one. Removal of chronic, nonfunctional lead would also avoid potential mechanical and electrical interaction with the new lead.
- ICD or pacemaker lead can be removed using direct or indirect traction method. Laser sheath can be valuable in direct traction method as it can facilitate cutting of chronic binding sites.
- Upgrading from a single-chamber to a dual-chamber system is common. The additional lead can usually be inserted without great difficulty.

Perioperative Issues

The overall success of ICD therapy certainly also depends on the balance of benefits over risk of its implantation procedure. To minimize the risk, all perioperative clinical and technical variables must be evaluated. In addition to the patient arrhythmia history, the underlying cardiac and overall clinical status are important perioperative parameters. The status of underlying LV function, as expected, is a strong predictor of outcome and although its influence is more evident in the thoracotomy approach (Tables 4-1 and 4-2), it should always be considered in the overall equation.

In the years of epicardial ICD system, the need for other cardiac operations, such as CABG, valvular replacement, or VT surgery, posed somewhat of a dilemma. On the one hand, the concomitant cardiac procedure would provide a technical advantage, but on the other hand, the combined operation would pose some limitation on defibrillation testing and overall would carry an increased surgical morbidity and mortality rate. Thus, in most cases, the physician would elect to apply the epicardial leads during the open chest surgical procedure and perform defibrillation testing and generator implantation at a later date. Consequently, it would not be uncommon to encounter the need to implant additional leads (such as a superior vena cave coil and/or an endocardial sensing lead) because of suboptimal performance of the empirically implanted epicardial system. With the advent of transvenous approach, there is no such dilemma. In addition, the simpler ICD implantation carries a very low risk.

With transvenous ICD implantation, the preoperative technical evaluation should include anatomical and physiological factors for lead passage and implantation. Thus, the status of venous patency, tricuspid valve, and right ventricular myocardial viability should be assessed. Patients with pre-existing ICD or pacemaker leads may pose difficulties with lead passage. These patients may require explantation of their pre-existing leads. Patients with right ventricular myocardial infarction, severe cardiomyopathy, and infiltrative diseases such as giant-cell myocarditis and sarcoidosis may create difficulties in obtaining adequate sensing and pacing.

It is also important to evaluate the possible need for catheter ablative therapy in patients undergoing transvenous ICD implantation because of potential difficulty in catheter placement posed by the indwelling ICD leads and the risk for lead dislodgment, especially the atrial lead. The common concomitant arrhythmias that are amenable to catheter ablation are AV nodal reentrant tachycardia, atrial tachycardia, and atrial flutter. Another common indication for catheter ablative procedure is poor rate control with paroxysmal atrial fibrillation. The typical ICD patient usually has a moderate or severe underlying LV dysfunction and therefore, can not tolerate many AV nodal blocking drugs. Consequently, episodes of paroxysmal atrial flutter or fibrillation may interfere with appropriate VT therapy even with activation of discriminatory criteria. Such a patient may be best managed with an AV nodal ablation.

Perioperative Mortality and Morbidity

With epicardial system implantation, operative morbidity is high and the procedure was even associated with moderate degree of mortality.[16-19] These adverse events can not be attributed only to the ICD procedure. Many patients undergoing ICD implantation in the past also had concomitant high-risk procedures, such as VT surgery and CABG, and valvular repair or replacement. The perioperative mortality reported in the literature ranged from 3 to 9%, which would be considered unacceptably high at current standard. In our institution, of the 85 patients undergoing AICD implantation without other high-risk cardiac surgical procedure between 1985-1989, there were three deaths (3.5%); two from sepsis and one from incessant VT/VF. Perioperative morbidity with the epicardial system was also high, with many postoperative complications involving mostly pulmonary issues, pericarditis, and concomitant arrhythmias. Atrial fibrillation was a common occurrence, especially in the first 48 hours after surgery. For this reason, it was prudent to keep the ICD inactive during the recovery period in the Intensive Care Unit.

Without the thoracotomy procedure, ICD implantation was associated with much lower perioperative mortality and morbidity. Reported overall mortality was in the order of 1%, and was even much lower in patients without significant underlying left ventricular dysfunction (NYHA Class I-II or LVEF > 30%).[20,21]

Table 4-1. Operative Mortality of Thoracotomy ICD Lead Implantation

Reference	Patients	Mortality (%)
Lessmeier et al (Multicenter Data)	300	2.7
Winkle et al	270	4.6
Levine et al	218	9.6
Saksena et al (Telectronics/Guardian Data)	200	5.5
Fromer et al (European Multicenter Data)	102	3.9
Stanford Data Base (1985-1989)	85	3.5

This low rate was evident even in the early experience of transvenous ICD with abdominal placement of the generator. In our combined institutions (Stanford University and Kaiser Permanente Santa Theresa), there was only one operative death of the 190 patients undergoing such implantation. Clearly, then, ICD therapy became more accepted and, eventually, emerged as the preferred form of therapy.

Table 4-2. Operative Mortality Comparison of Thoracotomy and Transvenous Lead System

Reference	Thoracotomy	Transvenous
Zipes et al (Multicenter PCD Data)	4.1%	0.7%
Saksena (Multicenter Data)	4.2%	1.8%
LVEF < 30%	5.2%	2.1%
NYHA III & IV	7.7%	3.9%
Stanford Data Base	3.5%	0.5%

> **Perioperative mortality and morbidity of transvenous ICD implantation are significantly lower than those associated with thoracotomy approach**

Perioperative Anticoagulation Management

A common delayed complication is the development of pocket hematoma, especially in patients in whom anticoagulation must be immediately re-initiated. Therefore, in general, if clinical condition permits, anticoagulation should be restarted slowly. In those patients with high risk for thromboembolism and require early anticoagulation, intravenous heparin can be restarted but with meticulous attention to signs and symptoms of hematoma. Such a situation is indeed problematic and is definitely associated with a high rate of postoperative bleeding and hematoma. Based on our anecdotal experience, we prefer to use intravenous heparin over subcutaneous low-molecular weight heparin during the transition period to coumadin. In our practice, we would delay the administration of heparin for several hours and place pressure dressing and/or a sandbag over the wound for the first 12-24 hours. We would also restart oral anticoagulation slowly, avoiding loading dosages.

> **Anticoagulation in the perioperative period would significantly increase the risk for ICD pocket hematoma but in some situation, this dilemma can not be avoided and the best general measure must be carried on**

Prophylactic Antibiotic

The rate of infection with transvenous ICD implantation is low and is approximately similar to the rate of infection with pacemaker implantation procedure. In general, it is well within the reported rate of infection of elective procedure with primary wound closure of 2% (The National Research Council for Wound Classification). Because of this low rate of infection, there has been no systematic study of the most appropriate use of prophylactic antibiotic. Most guidelines of such use are based primarily on historical data. Rarely does the "routine" practice of an institution omit the use of antibiotic entirely because device implantation is a procedure where the risk of infection, albeit low, carries a high monetary and morbidity penalty. It is therefore a widely accepted practice that prophylactic antibiotic should consist of, at least, preoperative administration of oral or intravenous antibiotic to cover common skin flora, such as *Staphylococus aureus* and *Staphylococus epidermidis* (such as 1 gram of intravenous cephalosporin).[22-24] It is also common to use antibiotics for wound irrigation. Postoperatively, practices vary widely in their standard, from none to a few intravenous doses for 24 hours to a one-week coverage. Antibiotic administration can be provided in various ways. It is, of course, prudent to keep in mind that there is no substitute for good infection control surgical technique and practice.

> Due to limited data, there are no specific recommendations for the use of prophylactic antibiotic for ICD implantation and therefore, it is usually carried on in the same manner as in pacemaker implantation

Postoperative Care

The postoperative care for the patient undergoing transvenous ICD implantation does not differ too much from the standard of care of patients undergoing pacemaker implantation. The most important issue is to assure lead stability and allow for proper wound healing. Therefore, the patient should be bedrest, undergo continuous cardiac monitoring, and be observed for pocket bleeding or hematoma. A chest X-ray is obtained to confirm the stability of lead(s) position and the absence of pneumothorax. Morbidity rate from ICD implantation using current technique is also very low.

The most common immediate clinical problem is pneumothorax from subclavian venous puncture, which occurs in 1-3% of cases. This complication is more common in the elderly patients. Its occurrence can usually be predicted by the degree of difficulty in cannulating the subclavian vein during the procedure. Its presence is easily noted at postoperative chest X-ray. Hence, if pneumothorax is suspected or anticipated, serial chest X-rays should be obtained; at least one immediately after the surgery and one the following day. Of note, chest tube placement is not always necessary, because a small pneumothorax of less than 20% of lung volume rarely causes significant respiratory insufficiency. For this same reason, one can not assume that pneumothorax is not present simply from the absence of respiratory symptoms. An associated, but more troublesome complication is hemothorax, which usually occurs also as a result of difficult and complicated venipuncture whereby the artery is accidentally cannulated.

Pericardial effusion and tamponade also occurs very rarely, but can easily detected with an echocardiogram. Pericardial effusion is usually caused by RV or RA perforation and is more common with the use of active fixation lead with a screw-in mechanism, especially when the lead has to be repositioned multiple times. The ICD lead is potentially more risky than a pacemaker lead because the ICD defibrillator lead is larger and may also require a stiffer styllete and its screw protrudes longer. However, this has not been observed clinically. The elderly patient is also more susceptible to this complication. This complication poses more serious morbidity because of the dilemma in its management. The associated pericarditis frequently becomes somewhat protracted because of the relative contraindication for anti-inflammatory agents in the early period. Consequently, atelectasis and its associated morbidity such as pneumonitis and pleural effusion can occur.

Delayed complications include pocket hematoma and infection as discussed above. Unfortunately, because patients are routinely discharged from the hospital the day after their procedure, signs and symptoms of these complications usually occur after their discharge and are likely to escape detection.

Post Discharge Management

After the immediate recovery period, the patient should be instructed to limit the use of the affected extremity to avoid lead dislodgment and wound irritation. In most cases, recovery can be accomplished at home after an overnight hospitalization. Strenuous use of the affected arm is discouraged for at least several days and until the patient is re-evaluated in the outpatient clinic.

The current standard of practice of early hospital discharge does not allow for meaningful evaluation of chronic lead parameters. The "pre-discharge" ICD testing was a routine procedure in the past because the hospital recovery of patients undergoing thoracotomy implantation would typically be about seven to ten days, allowing for some, if not adequate inflammatory tissue recovery at the lead-tissue interface. Current ICD implantation procedure rarely requires more than a 24-hour hospital stay. Consequently, a "chronic" testing is usually performed after hospital discharge.

As in the case of a pacemaker, in order to program the device optimally, all electrophysiologic parameters must be measured. In the case of ICD, this would include the assessment of efficacy and safety of VT and VF therapies. As mentioned above, assessment of VT therapy is not commonly performed at the time of implantation and indeed, the chronic device testing offers better environment for this measurement. Unlike the surgical environment, which allows for limited time for testing and which is also likely to influence inducibility of VT, the chronic testing allows for a thorough and more appropriate non-invasive programmed stimulation (NIPS). This opportunity should be utilized to assess efficacy and safety of ATP and low-energy shock for cardioversion. In addition, reproducibility of DFT estimation should be assessed.

Postoperative management after an ICD implantation also includes assessment of device parameters and performance, including confirmation of DFT, hence it would be necessary to perform non-invasive electrophysiology testing at one month

---

The disadvantage of this delayed testing is the possibility of an unanticipated and, potentially, undetected problems with lead and device status. In the absence of automatic lead integrity performance and an adequate warning system, lead dislodgment may escape detection and, consequently, the assumed patient's safety can be significantly jeopardized. For this reason, a quick and simple device interrogation should be performed in the outpatient setting shortly after hospital discharge, such as at the time of clinic visit for wound check. This examination should include the assessment of sensing, which can be easily performed by visual analysis of the intracardiac EGM. A good EGM would indicate stable lead position and therefore a good likelihood for adequate sensing, pacing and defibrillation efficacy.

> - Perioperative care of the ICD patient includes routine cardiopulmonary monitoring and post-operative assessment of lead placement and stability. Perioperative morbidity and mortality with endocardial ICD are much lower than those encountered with thoracotomy approach.
> - Prophylactic antibiotic for ICD implantation is provided in the same manner as with pacemaker implantation. It should consist of at least pre-operative oral or intravenous antibiotic to cover common skin flora.
> - Postoperative bedrest for 24 hours is usually recommended.
> - Perioperative anticoagulation can be problematic, especially when immediate re-anticoagulation is mandatory. There is a significant rate of pocket hematoma in such situation.

References

1. Babbs CF, Yim GK, Whistler SJ, *et al.* Elevation of ventricular defibrillation threshold in dogs by antiarrhythmic drugs. Am Heart J, 1979;**98**(3):345-350.
2. Tacker WA, Jr., Niebauer MJ, Babbs CF, *et al.* The effect of newer antiarrhythmic drugs on defibrillation threshold. Crit Care Med, 1980;**8**(3):177-180.
3. Jung W, Manz M, Pfeiffer D, *et al.* Effects of antiarrhythmic drugs on epicardial defibrillation energy requirements and the rate of defibrillator discharges. Pacing Clin Electrophysiol, 1993;**16**(1 Pt 2):198-201.
4. Manz M, Jung W, and Luderitz B. Interactions between drugs and devices: experimental and clinical studies. Am Heart J, 1994;**127**(4 Pt 2):978-984.
5. Kuhlkamp V, Mewis C, Suchalla R, *et al.* Effect of amiodarone and sotalol on the defibrillation threshold in comparison to patients without antiarrhythmic drug treatment. Int J Cardiol, 1999;**69**(3):271-279.
6. Flaker GC, Tummala R, and Wilson J. Comparison of right- and left-sided pectoral implantation parameters with the Jewel active can cardiodefibrillator. The World Wide Jewel Investigators. Pacing Clin Electrophysiol, 1998;**21**(2):447-451.
7. Block M, Hammel D, Borggrefe M, *et al.* [Transvenous subcutaneous implantation technique of the cardioverter/defibrillator]. Herz, 1994;**19**(5):259-277.
8. Roelke M, O'Nunain SS, Osswald S, *et al.* Subclavian crush syndrome complicating transvenous cardioverter defibrillator systems [see comments]. Pacing Clin Electrophysiol, 1995;**18**(5 Pt 1):973-979.
9. Bhandari AK, Isber N, Estioko M, *et al.* Efficacy of low-energy T wave shocks for induction of ventricular fibrillation in patients with implantable cardioverter defibrillators. J Electrocardiol, 1998;**31**(1):31-37.
10. Hwang C, Swerdlow CD, Kass RM, *et al.* Upper limit of vulnerability reliably predicts the defibrillation threshold in humans. Circulation, 1994;**90**(5):2308-2314.
11. Shepard RK, Wood MA, Dan D, *et al.* Induction of ventricular fibrillation by T wave shocks: observations from monophasic action potential recordings. J Interv Card Electrophysiol, 1999;**3**(4):335-340.
12. Swerdlow CD, Ahern T, Kass RM, *et al.* Upper limit of vulnerability is a good estimator of shock strength associated with 90% probability of successful defibrillation in humans with transvenous implantable cardioverter-defibrillators. J Am Coll Cardiol, 1996;**27**(5):1112-1118.
13. Taneja T, Goldberger J, Parker MA, *et al.* Reproducibility of ventricular fibrillation characteristics in patients undergoing implantable cardioverter defibrillator implantation. J Cardiovasc Electrophysiol, 1997;**8**(11):1209-1217.

14.   Levy T, Walker S, and Paul V. Initial experience in the extraction of chronically implanted pacemaker leads using the Excimer laser sheath. Heart, 1999;**82**(1):101-104.

15.   Wilkoff BL, Byrd CL, Love CJ, *et al.* Pacemaker lead extraction with the laser sheath: results of the pacing lead extraction with the excimer sheath (PLEXES) trial. J Am Coll Cardiol, 1999;**33**(6):1671-1676.

16.   Fromer M, Brachmann J, Block M, *et al.* Efficacy of automatic multimodal device therapy for ventricular tachyarrhythmias as delivered by a new implantable pacing cardioverter- defibrillator. Results of a European multicenter study of 102 implants [see comments]. Circulation, 1992;**86**(2):363-374.

17.   Lessmeier TJ, Lehmann MH, Steinman RT, *et al.* Implantable cardioverter-defibrillator therapy in 300 patients with coronary artery disease presenting exclusively with ventricular fibrillation. Am Heart J, 1994;**128**(2):211-218.

18.   Levine JH, Mellits ED, Baumgardner RA, *et al.* Predictors of first discharge and subsequent survival in patients with automatic implantable cardioverter-defibrillators. Circulation, 1991;**84**(2):558-566.

19.   Winkle RA, Mead RH, Ruder MA, *et al.* Long-term outcome with the automatic implantable cardioverter- defibrillator. J Am Coll Cardiol, 1989;**13**(6):1353-1361.

20.   Zipes DP and Roberts D. Results of the international study of the implantable pacemaker cardioverter-defibrillator. A comparison of epicardial and endocardial lead systems. The Pacemaker-Cardioverter-Defibrillator Investigators. Circulation, 1995;**92**(1):59-65.

21.   Saksena S, Mehta D, Krol RB, *et al.* Experience with a third-generation implantable cardioverter-defibrillator. Am J Cardiol, 1991;**67**(16):1375-1384.

22.   Da Costa A, Kirkorian G, Cucherat M, *et al.* Antibiotic prophylaxis for permanent pacemaker implantation: a meta- analysis. Circulation, 1998;**97**(18):1796-1801.

23.   Hartstein AI, Jackson J, and Gilbert DN. Prophylactic antibiotics and the insertion of permanent transvenous cardiac pacemakers. J Thorac Cardiovasc Surg, 1978;**75**(2):219-223.

24.   Muers MF, Arnold AG, and Sleight P. Prophylactic antibiotics for cardiac pacemaker implantation. A prospective trail. Br Heart J, 1981;**46**(5):539-544.

CHAPTER 5

PATIENT MANAGEMENT

General Considerations

The management of patients after ICD implantation consists of continuous assessment of several simultaneous issues involving device's components and operation as well as the patient's arrhythmia and overall clinical status. The state and stability of device's hardware is particularly important to monitor in the first few days and weeks after implantation because afterwards, very little can be done to alter its status. The performance and appropriateness of the software and parameters, on the other hand, needs to be closely assessed throughout the life of the system. Analysis, interpretation, and adjustment of these parameters must be correlated to the patient's needs and clinical status.

In general, basic sensing and pacing performance can be assessed in a manner that is similar to analyzing permanent pacemaker parameters. Appropriate sensing, in the case of ICD, is extremely important and one key issue to keep in mind is that sensing problems will result in an erroneous performance in both bradycardia support and tachycardia therapy. Thus, oversensing and double sensing would result in brady-pacing inhibition and, possibly, erroneous triggering of tachycardia therapy. In terms of pacing, inadequate capture would potentially result in pulse deficit as well as ineffective antitachycardia pacing therapy. In ICD with dual-chamber pacing and sensing capability, atrial sensing is useful in the algorithm of tachycardia detection, in terms of distinguishing VT from supraventricular tachycardia. In this respect, having the dual-chamber feature as part of the ICD is more advantageous than having a separate dual-chamber pacemaker. However, the dual-chamber ICD is more complex and the programming of bradycardia parameters can pose limitations to the tachycardia parameters and vice versa. The complex interaction between the parameters would become more apparent in the programming of rate-responsiveness and maximum tracking rates.

Once the initial appropriate programming has been performed, the patient would not typically need intensive follow-up, assuming that no malfunction occurs and the patient does not receive frequent shocks. In the event of malfunction leading to frequent shocks, the management of the patient can become quite complicated. In addition to the usual arrhythmia evaluation, the patient must undergo thorough device testing and, not of least importance, recover from the physical and psychological trauma.

> **Inappropriate shocks due can be very traumatic to the patient, therefore it would be prudent to program ICD parameters appropriately**

Hence, the best follow-up management of the ICD patient is to meticulously evaluate all components of the underlying arrhythmias and device parameters, and to anticipate potentials negative interactions and malfunction. Routine office visits at regular intervals would be the minimum interface between the patient and clinician. To assure device integrity, many units now perform routine self-testing and are equipped with a warning mechanism to alert the patient should a significant malfunction occurs in the interim.[1] For example, in the GEM (Medtronic) and Prizm (CPI) units, such warning functions can be activated.

Confirmation of DFT can only be assessed by inducing VF and delivering a high-energy shock. Thus, at a reasonable chronic interval, between one to three months after implantation, the patient is advised to undergo "defibrillation testing", where VF is again induced and the submaximal shock is tested. During this testing, the efficacy of other therapy, such as ATP and low-energy shock, which are usually not fully evaluated during initial implantation, can also be tested. The full spectrum of inducible VT can also be assessed and "fine tuning" of device's setting can therefore be done. After this testing, the DFT is assumed to be stable and no further DFT testing is usually performed. Obviously, this conclusion is based on the assumption that all other influencing factors remain stable. The DFT can indeed change over time, in spite of apparent stable clinical status.[2]   Of particular importance is the influence of antiarrhythmic drug. If the patient is subsequently placed on an antiarrhythmic drug, re-testing of the DFT may be of value because such a drug, especially amiodarone, can significantly raise the DFT.[3-6] For better assurance, some experts suggested periodic testing of DFT[1], although the validity of such recommendation has not yet been verified.

> The DFT can not be assessed without inducing VF, hence it is normally confirmed only once, at one month after implantation

Even when all parameters remain stable and device function remains appropriate, ICD patients are still faced with physical, psychological, legal, and economical issues.[7-14]   These concerns, which include important potential interactions with environmental elements will be discussed in this chapter.

Basic Programming

Device programming was not an issue with the early models, where the function of the ICD was only to treat VT/VF using only one form of therapy, high-energy shock. In such a situation, when arrhythmia condition changes, there was no other choice but to replace the device with a more appropriate one. Tailoring device performance to the patient's changing arrhythmia status has been made easier with the development of "programmable" ICD, which offered programmable values for rate cut off and shock energy. With the incorporation of tier-therapy for tachyarrhythmia, a full spectrum dual-chamber bradycardia pacing, and detection enhancement features, the ICD has become a much more complicated device to program.

The first task faced by the clinician after the ICD has been implanted is programming the device appropriately. There are key items to be kept at high priority in this important step. The ICD was designed to be a life saving device to treat the cause of sudden death. Thus, at the least, the ICD must be programmed to appropriately treat VF. For this very reason, the highest zone in a tier-therapy device typically only allows shock as its form of therapy. The other important programming step, which remains difficult at times, is designing a safe and appropriate therapy for VT. This has become an important step because with the addition of tier-therapy feature, the VF zone is likely to be set at a higher value than when only a single zone is available. The management of "VT" must take into consideration that the arrhythmia detected within this zone can have widely variable hemodynamic effects. In some respect, the physician is almost immediately faced with the decision whether to program one or two VT zones. This task becomes even more difficult when the patient's clinical VT is unknown, which is not uncommon nowadays as ICD is frequently implanted without pre-operative electrophysiology testing.

Programming VF Zone and Therapy

Programming VF Zone as the Only Zone

Programming this basic zone as a single zone is simple but for that very reason, errors may occur. The device, in fact, is programmed to this single zone nominally. The nominal detection rate/CL, however, varies among the brands. For instance, it is set at 165 bpm (CPI), 188 ms (Medtronic), 167 bpm/360 ms (Ventritex), or 202 bpm/297 ms (ELA). The wide variation in the "nominal" value for this key parameter reflects the notion that there is no consensus on the most common rate for VF and the assumption that the clinician would likely reprogram it.

A few key considerations come into play in the selection of the appropriate value for this VF zone: (1) this zone is intended for the most serious tachyarrhythmia, (2) only shock therapy is available, and (3) no SVT discrimination is available. Thus, the clinician must consider the consequences of programming a low rate cut off value for this zone because there is no mechanism for rejecting sinus tachycardia or atrial fibrillation and that all tachyarrhythmias will be treated with a shock, even if it were hemodynamically tolerated. For these reasons, programming the tachyarrhythmia zone to a single VF zone is most appropriate for patients with VF as the only or primary arrhythmia and the rate cut off should be programmed well above the maximum sinus rate. In the young and otherwise healthy patient, such rate cut off frequently must be programmed above 200/min. This high rate cut off would also be appropriate in such a patient because typically VT is not part of the spectrum of tachyarrhythmia. In the patient with underlying structural heart disease, it would be advisable to program a lower rate cut off or to add a VT zone empirically because there is a higher likelihood for the occurrence of unanticipated VT. Furthermore, such a patient would be less likely to be able to withstand VT for long duration. In this situation, it should be kept in mind that the relatively low rate cut off may be exceeded by ventricular rates during atrial fibrillation; hence effort must be taken in providing adequate AV blockade.

Programming detection to a VF-only zone must take into consideration that SVT discrimination is not available in this zone, thus the rate cut off must be programmed above the maximum sinus rate and maximum ventricular rate during atrial fibrillation

---

Programming therapy in this scenario should obviously be based on the data of DFT testing. Shock energy should be programmed to a value that would provide sufficient margin of safety. In carrying on the tradition from the older ICD models with monophasic waveform, it would be necessary to program the energy at 10 or 15 joules above the "DFT". If only minimum DFT testing is performed with two attempts at, typically, 20 joules, the maximum energy would be the only and natural choice for this zone. However, if a more meticulous testing is performed, the DFT could be estimated at a lower value between 5 and 15 joules (see also Chapter 4). Thus the first shock therapy for VF could be programmed to as low as 15 joules. In fact, a 5 joule margin of safety has been considered sufficient[15] and hence, if a value of less than 5 joules is estimated to be the DFT, the shock therapy can be programmed to as low as 10 joules. The ability to program a significantly lower shock therapy may have substantial clinical advantages. Primarily, the advantage is in the time required to charge to that energy level, and the incremental difference may be in the order of three to five seconds. Such a time difference may be enough to prevent the patient from experiencing full syncope from the tachyarrhythmia.

The subsequent shock therapies should be programmed to full energy because there is no clinical or technical advantage of using energy of an intermediate level. In fact, the delay from the first failed shock would have resulted in a prolonged VF duration, which would best treated with a maximum energy shock.

Programming VF Zone as Part of A Tier-Therapy Scheme

With the availability of tier-therapy, VF is commonly programmed as the highest zone in a multi-zone scheme. In this situation, it would be most advantageous to set the VF detection rate cut off to a higher value to broaden the range for the VT zone. It would not be uncommon to encounter ATP-responsive monomorphic VT at rates above 200 bpm, especially in patients who are not on any antiarrhythmic drug. If the zone of VT needs to include rates that are faster than 250, however, it would be advisable to program it using some discriminatory criteria to avoid delaying therapy for VF (see below under VT Programming Section and Dual-Chamber Algorithm Sections).

Programming VT Zone and Therapy

Programming VT Detection Zone(s)

There are many items to be considered in programming the VT zone(s) and therapies. Many of the new features of tier-therapy and arrhythmia discrimination apply mostly to the programming of the VT zone. To take full advantage of these features, both detection and therapy parameters must be programmed in such a way that would fit general principles and specific conditions of the patient's normal and abnormal rhythms. Some of the advanced features will be discussed in the next section of this chapter.

The detection window width must be programmed reasonably. It should be reasonably broad (e.g. greater than 20-30 bpm range) as to accommodate some variation in VT rate. However, a single VT zone should not be too large (e.g. covering a greater than 100 bpm range) because it would be difficult to program one type of therapy scheme that would be appropriate for all VT types with markedly different rates. For example, a therapy scheme that includes multiple ATP attempts would be appropriate for a VT with a rate of 130 bpm but not for one with a rate of 230 bpm. If the clinical situation requires such broad coverage, it would be more advisable to program two VT zones. In such a scheme, the lower zone would allow for a greater liberty for delaying shock. The hemodynamic status during VT in the lower-rate zone can usually tolerate more attempts of ATP. In contrast, the overall cardiovascular status during VT in the higher-rate zone may not tolerate more than a few ATP attempts. The potential adverse effects of prolonged hemodynamic compromise should be considered, including failure of back-up shock therapy.[16] In some units (Ventritex), there is a safety feature, the Extended High Rate (EHR), that can be programmed to prevent prolonged delay of shock therapy. The EHR is more direct method of determining the amount of time that would be allowed for less aggressive therapy such as ATP. The EHR timer is programmable from 10 seconds to five minutes. The CPI units are also equipped with such a safety feature, known as the ATP Time Out.

> **Having VT zones would allow implementation of SVT discriminatory features and ATP therapy, which are useful when the tachyarrhythmia detection zone is programmed at a low cut-off rate**

Having two VT zones would also allow for programming one zone at a very high rate, such as 250 bpm, especially when a safety feature is available. In the Medtronic units, this safety feature is available by programming the "Fast VT (FVT) via VF" method. With this scheme, fast monomorphic VT can be distinguished from fast polymorphic VT or VF because the latter would be more likely to have greater R-R interval variation that would result in crossing over to the VF zone.

In the CPI units, the "Shock When Unstable" feature can be utilized in the higher-rate VT zone if there is a concern that such a zone would overlap with polymorphic VT or slow VF. This feature is designed as a safety and can be used to implement shock (rather than ATP) therapy in such a case. This "Shock When Unstable" feature is not available in the lower-rate zone and, therefore, it would not interfere with the mode for distinguishing VT from AF, whereby the unstable R-R would activate the "Inhibit When Unstable" mode.

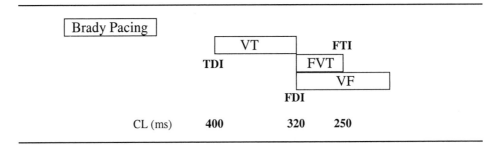

Figure 5-1. An example of a "Fast VT via VF" scheme, allowing programming of a VT zone with cycle lengths as short as 250 ms, yet with the safety feature of an overlapping VF zone

Programming VT Therapy

Anti Tachycardia Pacing Therapy

With respect to therapy, ATP feature has been found to be useful for VT. Most patients would experience minimal or no symptom from this form of therapy. Those who have experienced both ATP and shock therapies can greatly appreciate this advantage. Even patients who have not had any therapies from their ICD would be more reassured with the knowledge that the ICD would first attempt with a "less painful" type of therapy. The physician should also keep in mind that avoiding shock therapy also has other physical and psychological advantages. It would likely avoid any appreciable loss of consciousness, interruption of concentration and embarrassment. ATP therapy would also use less energy, which may, in turn impact on the overall device longevity.

Despite having such potential advantages, ATP is not commonly programmed, especially in patients with no clinical documentation of sustained monomorphic VT. Many physicians are concerned with the potential harm of programming ATP without knowing the patient's VT response to such therapy and the possibility of causing degeneration of the rhythm into VF. Although ATP certainly has the potential of accelerating a slow VT into a faster one, its efficacy has also been overlooked. Several studies have shown the efficacy and safety of programming ATP, even if it were done empirically.[17-20] Schaumann et al [20] found that even in patients with a diagnosis of only VF, VT was the arrhythmia in 85% of all tachyarrhythmia episodes and that ATP was successful in terminating the VT in 90% of cases, with 5.7% incidence of acceleration.

> **Antitachycardia pacing therapy, a painless form of therapy for VT, is a desirable alternative to shock and therefore should be utilized in the VT zone**

Programming the appropriate scheme of ATP may indeed be challenging. In principle, the key for achieving successful termination for VT is delivering the stimulus with sufficient prematurity within the excitable gap of the reentry circuit such that it depolarizes the excitable tissue and terminate the tachycardia by rendering it refractory.[21] Clearly, the success of this maneuver depends on several electrophysiological and clinical factors. One such factor is the size of the excitable gap, which is not readily known but can sometimes be inferred by the rate of the tachycardia. It has been noted that VT cycle length, as expected, plays an important factor in the success of ATP.[22-24] It was shown in these studies that ATP has lower efficacy and higher incidence of acceleration for VT with a rate of greater than 200-220 bpm. In this respect, antiarrhythmic drugs that slow conduction may offer a beneficial effect. Conversely, any factor that enhances conduction, such as cathecolamine, may narrow the gap and render the VT more difficult to terminate. It has been observed that circadian variation, perhaps as a reflection of the degree of cathecolamine, has an influence on the success of ATP; causing a higher incidence of VT acceleration in the early morning period.[25] The other critical factor that influences that success of ATP is the ability to deliver the stimulus with sufficient prematurity. This factor, in turn, is influenced by multiple electrophysiological properties. While many factors can not be altered, one factor, i.e. stimulus timing, is easily controlled and adjustable. While such timing can not be accurately measured in all instances, it can be estimated from the tachycardia cycle length. Thus, the stimulus (S1) is typically programmed at 20-50 ms or 10-20% shorter than the VT cycle length initially.

One important factor to keep in mind is the fact that the source of pacing during ATP is typically at a site very remote to the VT "focus". Thus, even when pacing coupling interval (CI) is set at (typically) 80% - 90% of the VT cycle length, the 10% - 20% prematurity only applies to the site of pacing. Multiple factors influence the delivery of this prematurity to the VT site. One factor is that the pacing site is typically very late into the VT cycle length (Figure 5-2), thus, the first few beats would not be effective at entraining the VT. This is evident in the varying degree of fusion noted in these early beats. Another factor is the distance between the site of pacing and the VT site, and conduction between those two sites.[26] Finally, another critical factor is the size of the excitable gap of the reentry, which was discussed earlier. Programming ATP must take these issues into consideration.

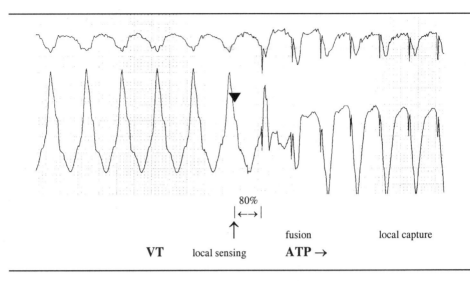

Figure 5-2. The onset of fixed-CI ("burst") ATP scheme in a patient with a slow VT of 400 ms CL. The ATP was programmed with an R-S1 prematurity of 80% (%RR). Even at this short CI, the first beat only minimally influenced the QRS configuration. This apparent delay is caused by late detection of VT at the pacing site (arrow), due to the fact that the pace/sense site (at the RV apex) was remote from the VT site LV lateral wall. Onset of local sensing is estimated from the first paced beat. The subsequent beats remain fused and complete local capture did not occur until the fourth beat. In this example, eight or more pacing pulses would be necessary to influence the VT site.

The critical degree of prematurity is achieved faster with a mode whereby the interval between each pacing stimulus is decremented ("ramp" or "auto-decremental" pacing, Chapter 3 & Figure 5-3). With such a mode, three to five stimuli may be sufficient. When using a mode with a constant interval between each stimulus ("burst" and "scan"), a greater number of stimuli, such as eight or ten, would probably be necessary. Furthermore, repeated stimulation at the site of slow conduction is also instrumental in the generation of conduction block and refractoriness in the mechanism of tachycardia termination. Thus, a longer burst is potentially also more advantageous than a shorter one. However, such estimation may be inaccurate and therefore, several attempts of ATP schemes should be implemented to increase the chance to be effective.

Success rates with the various types of ATP schemes have been compared and the results have so far been heterogeneous. In some reports, "burst" ATP was found to be more effective while in others, "ramp" was found to have the advantage.[24,27] If it is assumed that failure of a single ATP attempt is due to inadequate degree of stimulus prematurity with respect of the tachycardia cycle length, subsequent attempts should be applied using increasingly shorter coupling intervals ("scan"). However, some VT may not respond to ATP at all[28] and at some point, pacing attempts would involve a very short coupling interval and risk the induction of a more rapid tachycardia.[29] Unfortunately, the exact point of diminishing return in each instance is unknown, but it is recommended that the CI should not be allowed to go below 200 ms. In addition, there are data indicating that there would be no significant incremental advantage in programming more than four attempts of ATP.[30]

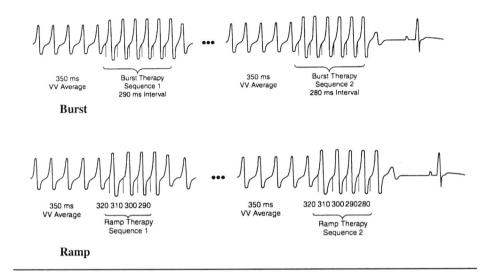

Figure 5-3. The difference between "burst" and "ramp" is shown, illustrating the effect of using decrementing coupling interval within a group of pacing (Reproduced with permission from Medtronic).

> **Due the heterogeneous nature of VT, ATP can rarely be tested accurately; hence, this form of therapy is usually programmed empirically, with the general goal of delivering repetitive stimuli with increasing prematurity as to influence the reentry site and terminate the VT**

A feature in Medtronic GEM models, the "SMART" mode, maybe useful in empiric programming of ATP. This feature keeps track of the result of ATP therapy and can assist in abandoning that therapy if it turns out to be ineffective in successive trials. When activated, the SMART mode would "skip" a therapy scheme that had failed four consecutive episodes, and as a result the ICD would deliver the next programmed therapy. For example, in the case that the last four consecutive VT episodes were not successfully terminated by Rx-1 (e.g. three "burst" attempts), Rx-2 (e.g. three "ramp" attempts) would be the first therapy for the next episode of VT. Hence, in the event that an empirically programmed ATP turns out to be ineffective, this mode would note and eliminate it.

Low-Energy Cardioversion Therapy

Another therapy for VT is low-energy cardioversion. This form of therapy was recognized as a potential therapy for VT because clinical experienced has shown that VT may respond to a shock with an energy that is lower than that used for VF. It was later tested and found to be effective in only approximately half of patients tested. A correlation was found with VT cycle length.[31,32] Low-energy cardioversion was found to be more effective for slower VT. In some of the effective cases, a very low energy was sufficient; producing much less discomfort when compared to full-energy shock. This method was later applied to the ICD and was considered potentially useful, especially within a tier-therapy scheme. In one prospective crossover study, Bardy et al, found a 63 % efficacy of auto-decrementing ATP scheme with 7-10 stimuli up to four attempts and 75 % efficacy of low-energy cardioversion with 0.2-2.0 joules also up to four attempts.[33] They also found similar rates of acceleration between ATP (17 %) and cardioversion (21 %). Saksena et al, in a similar randomized, prospective, crossover study, also found comparable efficacy of ATP (80%) and cardioversion (83%) as well as incidence of acceleration (6% and 11%, respectively).[34]

There are several disadvantages of low-energy cardioversion. It has been associated with a risk of inducing VF. Acceleration of VT into VF can occur at any energy level, even at less than one joule. The incidence of acceleration has been observed to be as high as 35%.[31,35,36] In our study [36], we found that patients with poor left ventricular function were at particularly high risk for VT acceleration with low-energy cardioversion. Furthermore, at energy levels above one joule, it is frequently perceived to be as painful as full-energy shock. Finally, low-energy cardioversion uses more energy than ATP. When all of these issues are considered, low-energy cardioversion is probably most useful as a back up to ATP. Ideally, its efficacy safety in each case should be determined. Following low-energy cardioversion, the therapy should be high-energy shock, at a value similar to the one programmed for VF.

> **Although low-energy cardioversion may have similar efficacy as ATP, it is usually more painful and therefore offers little advantage to the patient**

> - In programming a single zone ("VF") note that the nominal rate cutoff is not uniform and is frequently slow (e.g.165 bpm) and that detection enhancement can not be activated.
> - Using tier-therapy allows for ATP, low-energy CV and SVT discrimination. Programming two VT zones allows for more ATP schemes as well as overlapping zones (FVT in Medtronic models) for VT with short coupling intervals such as 250 ms.
> - ATP efficacy is difficult to assess and can be programmed empirically, even in patients with no documented VT. Burst and ramp modes are probably equally effective.
> - Low-energy CV is usually just as painful as high-energy shock. Its efficacy and risk for acceleration are probably equal to ATP.

Utilizing Detection Enhancement Features

Detection enhancement features are designed to improve discrimination between VT and supraventricular tachyarrhythmias. The first features were designed to equip single-chamber ICD. Hence, with only single-chamber information available, the most useful features were those related to typical characteristics of VT, such as its sudden onset, R-R stability, and width of the electrogram. Although these detection enhancement features appear to be simplistic, it was useful in differentiating VT from the most common supraventricular rhythms, sinus tachycardia and atrial fibrillation. Obviously they would not be useful in distinguishing VT from other tachyarrhythmia with sudden onset and regular R-R interval such as atrial flutter and AV nodal reentrant tachycardia. In such cases, the width or morphology feature maybe more advantageous.

With dual-chamber ICDs, the atrial channel provides a critical additional information and, in theory, can facilitate more accurate differentiation between VT and SVT. The incorporation of dual-chamber information into the algorithm is different and unique to each manufacturer's model.

Programming Onset and Stability Criteria

There has not been a general consensus on the exact or most appropriate values of onset and stability criteria. In several analyses, a significant overlap was noted between VT and SVT in terms of the onset and stability, and hence, sensitivity would always be jeopardized by attempts at improving discrimination. It is not surprising that a wide range of values were used in the several published reports. In an analysis of CPI devices' stored electrograms of 253 episodes of tachyarrhythmia (201 VT and 52 atrial arrhythmias), Neuzner noted a range of onset and stability overlaps between VT and atrial arrhythmias.[37] In terms of onset, to preserve a sensitivity of VT detection at > 95%, a 31% or greater onset criterion was needed, which provided only a 39% degree of specificity. The R-R stability provided a better discrimination. A stability value of < 24 ms gave a 71% specificity while still maintaining a greater than 97% sensitivity. In this report, however, all atrial arrhythmias were grouped as a single entity; hence the intended specificity for each of the criterion (onset for sinus tachycardia and stability for AF) could not be addressed. Brugada et al[38] specifically analyzed the utility of these criteria for differentiating VT (497 episodes) from sinus tachycardia (67 episodes) and atrial flutter/fibrillation (94 and 32 episodes, respectively) in 82 consecutive patients with CPI devices. They noted that VT was markedly different from sinus tachycardia in terms of its R-R interval change at onset (32% vs 2%) and from AF in terms of R-R stability (16 ms vs 49 ms). Similarly, in an analysis of 641 VT episodes in 150 patients, Schaumann et al[39] noted that > 96% of VT episodes had an onset value of > 9% and a stability value of < 30 ms). In their study of 100 patients, Swerdlow et al noted that an 87% onset ratio reduced detection of sinus tachycardia by 98% but caused underdetection of VT by 0.5%, while 40 ms stability criterion reduced detection of induced and paroxysmal AF by 95% and chronic AF by 99%.[40]

While there is probably no exact value for onset and stability that would be most "appropriate", the data indicate that 5-15% onset delta (85-95% onset ratio) and a 20-40 ms stability can be used without significantly jeopardizing VT detection. Using these values, these discrimination features achieve good specificity while maintaining adequate sensitivity for VT detection above 95%-99%.[38,40-42] To protect the patient from a potentially serious outcome in the event of VT under detection, safety net features, when available, should be employed. Such a safety net feature would activate therapy in the event that the tachyarrhythmia (of uncertain mechanism) persists for an extended time period. The time period (Sustained Rate Duration in CPI units) is programmable. The range for SRD is from 10 seconds to 60 minutes, allowing the physician to choose a value that is appropriate for specific circumstances. Thus, if the detection enhancement feature is to allow the patient to exercise to a relatively high heart rate, an SRD of 10-15 minutes may be appropriate. Conversely, if the zone includes very high rates, a shorter SRD, such as 30 to 60 seconds may be more appropriate.

Programming QRS Width or Morphology

Although these two features are significantly different in their method of implementation, they use a similar concept, based on the assumption that the ventricular electrogram (EGM) of VT would be different from that of supraventricular origin. The EGM width criterion, which uses far field signal, takes advantage of the idea that such a signal is more global and, like the surface ECG, would likely to detect a wide "QRS" complex during VT. The "width" is measured between the onset and offset of the electrogram, which are determined by the (programmable) slew rate thresholds (Figure 3-20). The EGM width criterion can be programmed to "active", "passive", or "off". In the "passive" mode, the EGM width will be measured but not used to withhold therapy, which offers a convenient way to obtain baseline data for potential use of the feature. The EGM width during baseline sinus rhythm was noted to fluctuate but stabilize after six months[43,44], at 60 to 72 ms, and not influenced by increase in heart rate [45]. However, it can be increased by antiarrhythmic drug (procainamide) [45] and artificially altered by exercise [46], especially within the first six months after implantation [44].

The EGM width criterion is valuable in further lowering the incidence of inappropriate therapy. In a study of 17 patients who had inappropriate detection of sinus tachycardia and atrial fibrillation, the addition of EGM width criterion to decreased the incidence of inappropriate detection using Onset and Stability alone from 36% to 5% and from 12% to 2%, respectively.[44] Based on the few clinical studies available, the EGM width should be programmed at a value above the width during sinus rhythm, typically at 75-80 ms, and the slew threshold should be programmed at a low value of 40-50 mV/s. The data from measurement during sinus rhythm would help this estimation. The EGM width criterion has less value in patients with an underlying wide QRS complex such as left bundle branch blocks.

> **The EGM Width criterion should ideally be programmed based on measured parameters during sinus rhythm (which can be obtained from data acquired during the "passive" mode); alternatively, the recommended values can be used**

The EGM Morphology Discrimination (MD) criterion is principally different from the EGM width. It uses a template that is acquired during baseline rhythm and compares it to the EGM during tachycardia. Thus, this feature does not rely only on a change in the width of the electrogram, and would have the advantage of being able to distinguish a wide-complex VT from a wide-complex SVT with aberrancy. In a study performed by the manufacturer, this criterion was shown to have 78.7% specificity while maintaining a 99.4% sensitivity. Another study performed with the Angstrom ICD that analyzed 216 spontaneous tachyarrhythmia episodes, also yielded a high sensitivity of 98% and a specificity of 80% using 60% match as the cut off.[47] The failure to detect VT/VF occurred with the parameter programmed to the "passive" mode. These values were comparable to the specificity and sensitivity achieved by the PR Logic algorithm using dual-chamber information.

In a study of 15 patients, the Morphology Discrimination feature has been shown to be reliable during increase in heart rate by pacing o exercise, as well as during atrial fibrillation with "matching" at greater than 80% in all three cases [48]. The challenge is to determine the appropriate degree of "match" that would accurately differentiate VT from SVT with the same goal of optimizing specificity and sensitivity. Clinical data on this feature suggest that a value between "60-80% match" would be optimal.

> **The Morphology Discrimination criterion, which offers some advantages over the EGM Width method, is typically programmed at "60-80% match" value**

> - There are no guidelines for the most appropriate values of onset and stability criteria. Data from several clinical studies indicate that 5-15% onset delta (85-95% onset ratio) and 20-40 ms stability yields good specificity while maintaining 95-99% sensitivity. If available, a safety net (SRD) should be used.
> - EGM width is typically programmed at > 75- 80 ms with a low slew rate of < 40-50 mV/s. The "passive" mode can be first programmed to collect data of EGM width during VT.
> - EGM Morphology Discrimination (MD) can be programmed to 60-80% match, which gives 80% specificity while maintaining 98% sensitivity. The "passive" mode would enable data collection to be used for more accurate "match".

Programming Detection Enhancement in Dual-Chamber ICDs

The addition of the atrial channel provides the possibility of comparing the atrial and ventricular channel activity in aiding the differentiation between VT and SVT. The incorporation of information from the atrial channel into the algorithm can be performed in many different ways. In this respect, each manufacturer has a different and unique method of rhythm analysis (see also Chapter 3). The programming of each of the algorithm will be discussed separately.

Programming CPI Dual-Chamber Algorithm

In the CPI units, information from the atrial channel is used in addition to the Onset and Stability criteria to prevent under detection of VT from these criteria. This is performed by assessing for the presence of atrial fibrillation and by comparing the atrial and ventricular (V) rates. Thus, VT rejection by the Stability criterion would be cross-checked by the "AFib Rate Threshold" value (programmable between 240-400 bpm) while VT rejection by Onset criterion would be cross-checked by the "V Rate > A Rate" assessment. The diagnosis of AF is made when the atrial rate is above the AF Rate Threshold value (programmable from 240-400 bpm) but only when the R-R is unstable. For this reason, atrial flutter with regular R-R interval would not likely be identified, even if the atrial rate exceeds the AF Rate Threshold. Other types of SVT, except for sinus tachycardia would also not be readily distinguished.

Programming the dual chamber algorithm in the CPI units involves choosing a value for the AF Rate Threshold, which is programmable between 240-400 bpm. The choice must obviously be determined based on the patient's clinical situation. To include atrial flutter, the lower value (e.g. 250 bpm) would be a good choice. Onset and Stability criteria must also be programmed, either as "Onset And Stability" or "Onset Or Stability". If "Onset Or Stability" is programmed, VT therapy would be initiated if either criterion is satisfied, which would improve sensitivity for VT detection but reduce specificity for SVT discrimination. If "Onset And Stability" is programmed, specificity would be increased. In such a case, the Sustained Rate Duration can be programmed as a safety net.

> Dual-chamber criteria in the CPI units, which is designed to prevent VT under detection from Onset and Stability criteria, is programmed by selecting an AFib Rate Threshold value

Programming Medtronic PR Logic™ Algorithm

To activate the PR Logic™ algorithm (Medtronic GEM products), the three components, AFib/AFlutter, Sinus Tach, and Other 1:1 SVTs, must be turned on. The SVT Limit value must also be selected. This value limits the shortest interval for the application of the detection enhancement. Tachycardia with R-R interval below this value would be treated as VT/FVT/VF, depending on which zone it falls. If the SVT Limit is programmed below the VF cut off rate (FDI), it would not apply for the portion with R-R interval below the FDI. The algorithm would also cross check for VT at all times. If AFib is noted but the R-R is stable (and is below SVT Limit), then double tachycardia is declared and the Double Tachycardia Detection algorithm is applied.

For AF to be declared, the requirements are: (1) median V interval must be between SVT Limit and TDI, (2) R-R instability (V CL regularity < 50%), (3) atrial median interval must be at least 6% faster than V, (4) AF Evidence Counter satisfied (Figure 5-4).

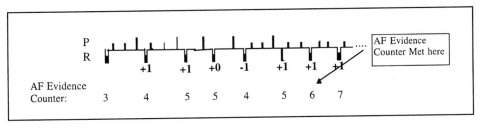

Figure 5-4. An example of AF Evidence Counter (Reproduced with permission from Medtronic).

For sinus tachycardia, the requirements are: (1) 1:1 A/V relationship with (2) the A falling in the antegrade zone (Figure 5-5).

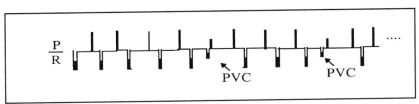

Figure 5-5. The typical pattern of sinus tachycardia (Reproduced with permission from Medtronic)

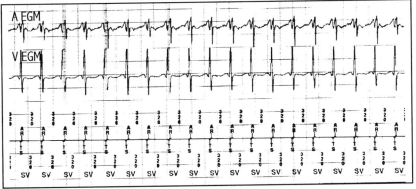

Figure 5-6. A typical pattern of SVT, such as AVNRT, with the A falling in the junctional zone of the V-V interval (Reproduced with permission from Medtronic).

In the latest report of the GEM DR worldwide study involving 497 patients, the algorithm (using SVT Limit of 320 ms), correctly classified 461/657 (70%) true SVT as SVT and all 1800 (100%) true VT/VF episodes as VT/VF. Misclassification of SVT as VT/VF was mainly due to 1:1 SVT with long AV delay and AF with short R-R below the SVT Limit or in the VF zone. The specificity was a 60% improvement from a single chamber system algorithm.[49,50] Similar results were noted from a European multicenter study involving 216 patients; showing 100% sensitivity and 71% specificity.[51]

In programming the PR Logic algorithm, those issues must be taken into consideration. A 1:1 SVT with long AV delay would have its atrial event falling in the retrograde zone of the V-V interval and be classified as VT (Figure 3-X). For the same reason, a VT with 1:1 but delayed V-A conduction would have its atrial event falling within the antegrade zone (second half) of the V-V interval and could therefore be classified as an SVT with 1:1 conduction. The potential for such misclassifications underscores the need for identifying the patient's baseline electrophysiologic profile.

> **The PR Logic algorithm, which provide an extensive assessment of A and V relationship, is programmed by activating the SVT criteria (AFib/Aflutter, Sinus Tach, and Other 1:1 SVTs) and selecting the SVT Limit value**

For the patient with a history of AF with rapid ventricular conduction, the nominal SVT Limit value of 320 ms may be too conservative. In such a case, the physician should make a clinical decision whether to upgrade the patient's therapy for AF rate control or to program the SVT Limit to a lower value. In some studies, programming the SVT Limit value to 250 ms was found to be beneficial in improving the specificity of the algorithm without jeopardizing sensitivity. In fact, in one study involving 47 patients, using a low SVT Limit of 240 ms and high TDI of 500 ms improved the specificity for SVT (90%), atrial fibrillation (78%), and sinus tachycardia (91%) while maintaining 100% sensitivity for VT/VF [52].

Programming Ventritex (St. Jude) Dual-Chamber Algorithm

The Ventritex (St. Jude) dual-chamber algorithm first places the rhythm into one of three categories depending on whether the V rate < A rate, the V rate = A rate, or the V rate > A rate. In the V<A Branch, the likely SVT rhythm would be AF, thus Morphology and/or Stability can be programmed. If not programmed, the rhythm would be assumed to be AF. In the V = A Branch, AV Interval is analyzed, and if dissociated, VT is diagnosed, while if it is associated (or not turned on), Morphology and/or Onset can be opted to distinguish VT from sinus tachycardia or other 1:1 SVTs. V>A Branch would automatically result in VT therapy.

The programmable steps are illustrated in Figure 5-7. These are Morphology, Stability, Onset, and AV Interval. The programmable steps include the basic criteria of Morphology, Onset, and Stability. These parameters have been discussed earlier. Thus, the respective values would still apply in this case. At the time of this publication, there has been no published data on the results of using this algorithm for SVT discrimination.

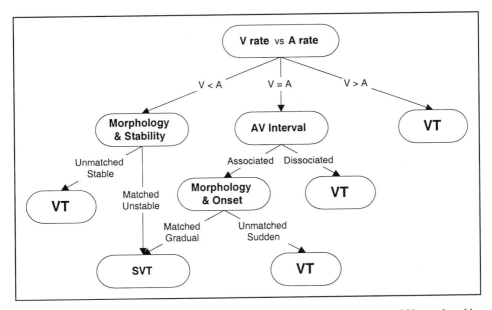

Figure 5-7. The Ventritex algorithm. The three branches (V<A, V=A, V>A) would be analyzed by steps that are programmable: AV Interval, Morphology, Stability, and Onset. The V=A Branch itself can be programmed OFF, in which case it would default to a VT diagnosis.

> **The dual-chamber algorithm in the Ventritex/St.Jude unit also utilizes the relationship between A and V and integrates Morphology, Onset and Stability criteria**

Programming ELA PARAD™ Dual-Chamber Algorithm

The ELA algorithm has always included the dual-chamber data. The algorithm uses Stability, PR Association, Acceleration (similar to Onset), and Origin of Acceleration criteria (Figure 3-25). Of importance is that the algorithm uses Stability as the first differentiating step. This is based on the notion that polymorphic VT is frequently self-terminating and that if it becomes a sustained episode, it would degenerate into VF. Otherwise it is noted that polymorphic VT still would have more R-R stability than rapidly conducted atrial fibrillation. The recommended value to program for Stability criterion is the nominal value of 63 ms. This is also the recommended value for the VT Long Cycle (VTLC) gap. This value is used to distinguish VT from pseudo-regular R-R tachycardia where there is no PR association, such as rapid AF with nearly regular R-R interval. This criterion uses only a single R-R variation instead of a window of R-R cycles (which must satisfy the programmed X of Y cycles of VT). The presence of a single VTLC it would declare the arrhythmia as AF or A Flutter and inhibit therapy (Figure 5-8).

ELA has been using its dual-chamber detection criterion for a few years. Early data involving a relatively small number of patients showed that this algorithm was excellent in differentiating SVT from VT (at 92% specificity) while preserving VT and VF detection at 100% for each.[53] Subsequent data confirmed these findings of good specificity (of 90.4%) and sensitivity (of 98.3%).[54]

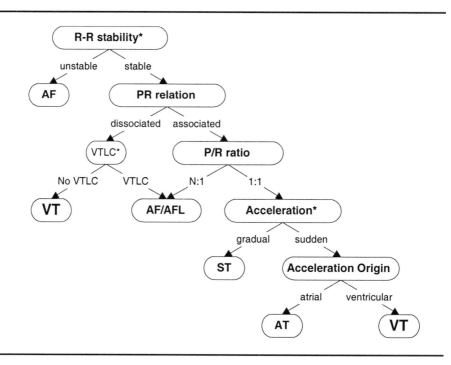

Figure 5-8. The PARAD algorithm illustrating the sequence of steps utilizing the Stability, PR association, VTLC, Acceleration, and Origin of Acceleration criteria. The asterisk indicates values that are programmable.

The results of the latest published study involving 82 patients showed that polymorphic VT could fall under the diagnosis of AF (occurring in one patient only). In that study, however, there was an excellent overall sensitivity of 98.5%, and specificity of 91.5%.[55] One of the SVT that was diagnosed as VT was atrial flutter with 2:1 regular ventricular conduction.

The accurate distinction between atrial and ventricular tachycardia may, in part be due to the unique feature of Origin of Acceleration. Using such a criterion, there would not be a confusion between an antegrade and retrograde atrial activation.

The programmable values in the PARAD™ are the Stability, VTCL, and the Acceleration. The Stability is programmable between 16 to 125 ms, with a nominal value of 63ms. The VTLC is programmable from 16 to 203 ms with a nominal value of also 63 ms (and a shipped value of 172 ms). The Acceleration is programmable from 6 to 50% fraction of the previous cycle, with a nominal value of 25%.

Programming PARAD algorithm requires the selection of Stability, VT Long Cycle, and Acceleration values and the nominal values (which were used in their clinical studies) are clinically reasonable as these have been shown to yield excellent specificity and sensitivity

---

Programming Biotronik SMART™ Dual-Chamber Algorithm

The Biotronik algorithm also uses AV relationship in addition to rate criterion. It assesses PP, RR, and PR intervals. Similar to Ventritex algorithm, the tachyarrhythmia is first classified into three categories: RR<PP, RR>PP, RR=PP.

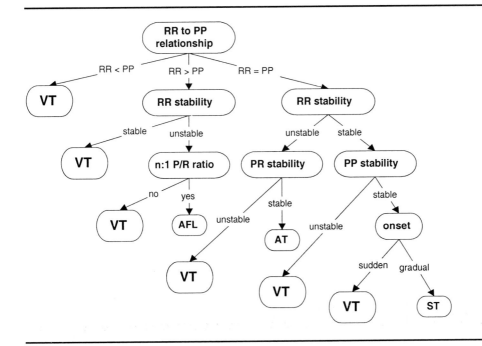

Figure 5-9. The SMART™ algorithm which starts with the three arms, RR<PP, RR>PP, and RR=PP. Subsequently Stability, Onset and PR relationship are integrated.

The algorithm uses the clinical assumption that the chamber with the higher rate is the origin of the tachycardia. However, the presence of VT is always monitored in the non-VT arms (RR>PP and RR=PP).

RR Stability is used to differentiate VT from SVT in the SVT (RR>PP) and RR=PP arms. The Stability value can be programmed programmed using absolute values (between 20 to 180 ms) or an "adaptive" value (between 5 to 30%) from the previous interval.

The Onset criterion is used late in the RR=PP arm's algorithm, for differentiation in the case of stable RR and PP intervals to differentiate between VT and sinus tachycardia. Programming Onset Delta can also be performed in one of two ways, using absolute values (between 30 to 500 ms) or "adaptive" value (between 10 to 90%) from the previous interval. As with other algorithms that rely on Onset to differentiate VT from SVT, the drawback at this step is that reentry atrial tachycardia (AT), AV nodal reentrant (AVNRT) or AV reciprocating tachycardia (AVRT), which usually also have a sudden onset, can not be differentiated.

> To program the SMART™ algorithm, values for Onset and Stability must be selected and based on preliminary data, the nominal values yield good specificity and sensitivity

An added "extrastimulus feature", which relies on the assumption that a premature beat from the chamber of tachycardia origin would advance the other chamber but not vice versa, is only useful in the distinction between VT and sudden-onset reentry AT. AVNRT and AVRT, which can conduct "PVC" rapidly, can still not be distinguished from VT using that method.[56] The SMART™ algorithm offers deletion of this step if it is known that the patient does not have VA conduction during VT in which case a Stable R-R tachycardia with RR=PP would not likely be a VT. There are limited data on the performance of the SMART™ algorithm as the clinical study was only recently completed.

Overall Performance of Dual-Chamber Algorithm

Although all dual-chamber algorithms utilize the information from the atrial and ventricular channels for the same purpose of differentiating SVT from VT, each algorithm offers its unique features that may be advantageous in certain conditions. The PR-Logic™ algorithm is probably more comprehensive than others in terms of its analysis of A-to-V association but other algorithm, such as the PARAD™ offers clinically useful features, such as the assessment of the origin of tachycardia. The Ventritex/St.Jude PHOTON's algorithm is, in general, similar to the Biotronik's SMART™ algorithm in terms of categorizing the tachycardia based on the comparison of RR to PP count, but the PHOTON features Morphology Discrimination that is unique to Ventritex models. The actual advantage of these unique features can not be assessed systematically because there would be no mechanism for comparing one to another. In fact, there has been no definitive data on the advantages of dual-chamber algorithm over single-chamber criteria. From published clinical data, there appears to be improvement in SVT discrimination from an overall specificity of 70%-80% to the 90% range. However, the actual improvement would not be known until completion of currently ongoing clinical trials addressing this issue specifically.

- Programming detection enhancements in dual-chamber ICD must be individualized to the patient and the features specific to the unit.
- In CPI Atrial-View, the AFib Rate (programmable between 240-400 bpm) should be selected based on the patient's atrial arrhythmia rate (e.g. 250). Onset and Stability must also be programmed, as "Onset And Stability" or "Onset Or Stability".
- For Medtronic PR Logic, the three SVT discriminations (AFib/Flutter, Sinus Tach, and Other 1:1 SVTs) can be activated individually. An SVT Limit (cycle length) value must then be selected. Data from clinical studies indicate that a value of 240-250 ms provided 80-90% specificity while maintaining 100% sensitivity.
- For Ventritex Photon, values for Morphology match, Onset, and Stability must be programmed. Data are limited so far.
- For ELA PARAD, three parameters must be programmed, Stability (nominal 63 ms), VT Long Cycle (nominal 63 ms), and Acceleration (nominal 25%). Limited data showed that the nominal values yielded good specificity (92%) and excellent sensitivity (99%).
- For Biotronik SMART, Stability and Onset must be programmed. Limited data showed nominal values provided good specificity and sensitivity.

Programming Bradycardia Parameters

With respect to bradycardia support, the pacemaker of an ICD functions in much the same way as a standard bradycardia device. Therefore, many of the steps in programming would not be reviewed. It would be important, however, to note that not all ICD models bradycardia pacemaker function have the secondary features, such as rate responsiveness and mode switch/conversion. The potential need for such features must be considered before making the choice of a specific ICD model.

The parameters of the pacemaker of an ICD-pacemaker combination device may, however, affect the operation of its tachycardia detection. These conflicting issues are relatively minor and noted more in patients who need frequent bradycardia support and experience episodes of slow VT.

Bradycardia and Tachycardia Rate Conflict

One such conflict involves a basic parameter, the pacing and detection rate. In all models except for ELA Defender, the zone of bradycardia can not overlap with the tachycardia detection zone. Such a dilemma, although rarely encountered, can be clinically significant. A typical scenario is the patient with a slow VT. With most ICD units, when the VT zone has to be programmed down to, for example, a rate of 130 bpm, the highest pacing upper sensor and tracking rates can not be programmed above 120 bpm (Figures 5-10). There is usually a distinct separation between the highest programmable upper tracking/sensor rate and the lowest VT detection zone rate (Table3-2).

Thus, even though the maximum upper rate limit can be programmed to high values such as 175 bpm (maximum tracking and sensor rates in CPI) or 185 bpm (maximum tracking rate in Biotronik models), in most cases it is limited by the VT zone. Typically, it can be programmed only up to 5-10 bpm below the VT detection zone. In some units, the maximum possible programmable value may be relatively low, such as at 120 bpm in the Medtronic GEM and furthermore, some models are still not equipped with rate responsiveness (CPI Mini and some AV models, Ventritex Countour & Profile models, and Biotronik Phylax).

With the exception of ELA's Defender, the upper tracking and sensor pacing rate limit in ICD units can not exceed the lowest tachycardia detection zone

---

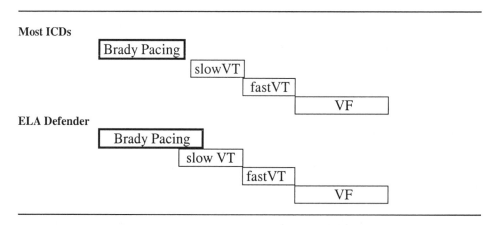

Figure 5-10. An illustration of the non-overlapping and overlapping of the bradycardia and tachycardia zones.

Refractory and Blanking Periods

As described earlier (Chapter 3), to avoid over-sensing, refractory periods are implemented, during which a signal would not be integrated into bradycardia or tachycardia analysis. Such signal would not inhibit bradycardia pacing and would not be included into tachyarrhythmia pulse count. This feature has great clinical significance in the ICD because the consequence of oversensing could result in inappropriate and unnecessary shock. On the other hand, this feature can also cause underdetection, which would also be detrimental with respect to tachyarrhythmia therapy. Most refractory periods are, therefore, typically short. The refractory period after a sensed ventricular event, which is implemented to avoid double counting is typically 8-130 ms. After a paced atrial event, ventricular refractory period to avoid cross talk is also short, at 30-50 ms. Such short refractory (blanking) periods are also therefore non-programmable.

The ventricular refractory period (VRP) after a paced ventricular event to avoid T-wave sensing is usually longer, and can range between 240-400 ms. Such a long refractory period can have adverse consequences. Consecutive ventricular tachyarrhythmia complexes can go undetected. Furthermore, if such a long refractory period occupies too much of the bradycardia-pacing interval, it may shorten the detection window such that VT may entirely escape detection. For those reasons, it is recommended that the refractory period after a paced ventricular event not be programmed to more than 50% of the pacing interval. This scenario limits the programming of both the refractory period and pacing rate. The CPI Prizm features Dynamic VRP, which shortens the VRP in dual-chamber devices to accommodate the narrowing of ventricular sensing window as ventricular pacing increases. A study testing this feature using 250 ms and 150 ms as the longest and shortest VRP during sensor-driven rate increase showed that the maintenance of large sensing window did not result in T-wave over-sensing.[57]

The atrial refractory periods can also cause similar problem with underdetection, although the consequences are not clinically serious. A long PVARP may cause underdetection of a premature atrial complex (PAC) and atrial tachyarrhythmias. Underdetection of a PAC can cause atrial pacing within the atrial vulnerable period, triggering an atrial arrhythmia. This can be avoided in Medtronic GEM by utilizing the Non-Competitive Atrial Pacing feature, which would delay atrial pacing by 300 ms after a sensed atrial complex within the PVARP. This feature is also available in CPI Prizm as Atrial Flutter Response, which would continue search for subsequent atrial event in multiple of intervals (programmable between 130-230 bpm) and would therefore avoid atrial pacing and trigger mode switch as well.

> The advantages and disadvantages in programming certain refractory period must be assessed in individual patients

Rate Smoothing and Ventricular Rate Stabilization Features

These features were designed to lessen the large variations of R-R interval that is caused by premature complexes. Such large variations do not only cause rhythm discomfort, they have also been implicated as the potential trigger to some ventricular tachyarrhythmias (the so-called "short-long-short" phenomenon).[58-60]

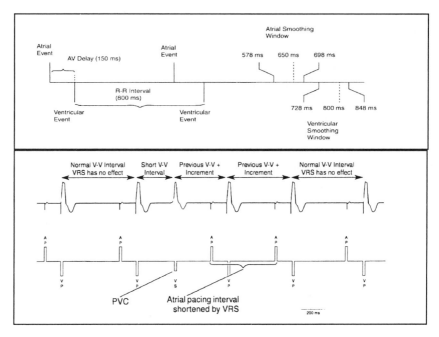

Figure 5-11. The operation of Rate Smoothing (CPI, top diagram) and Ventricular Rate Stabilization (Medtronic, bottom diagram) in the dual-chamber mode (Reproduced with permission from Guidant and Medtronic).

Both of these features adjust the pause following a premature complex to minimize the differences in R-R interval. The Rate Smoothing (CPI) is programmable as a percentage value while the Ventricular Rate Stabilization (Medtronic) is programmable in increment (that would be allowed to change from the previous coupling interval). These parameters can be programmed in both single- and dual-chamber ICD (Figure 5-11).

> **Rate Smoothing and Ventricular Rate Stabilization features may be useful in patients with frequent VT due to short-long-short interval**

Post-Shock Bradycardia Parameters

Because tissue and electrophysiologic properties after a high-energy shock may change significantly for a brief period of time, post-shock bradycardia pacing parameters are usually programmed differently. Of major concerns are the potentially more arrhythmogenic period immediately after a shock and the more refractory tissue for an extended period of time. Thus, typically, it would be advisable to delay the onset of bradycardia pacing and to program the pacing output values higher for a period of time to assure capture.

In CPI units, the post-shock pacing is operational after a high-energy shock; starting after a programmable interval (Post-Shock Pacing delay, 1.5-10 seconds) and for a programmable period of time (Post-Shock Pacing Period, 15 seconds to 60 minutes). In Medtronic units, it is operational starting at the start of charging period and lasts until one of the following events occurs: (1) episode termination, (2) 25 events after delivery of high-energy shock, (3) another therapy starts, or (4) high-energy therapy aborts. In Ventritex units, post-shock pacing is only delayed, by suppressing a programmable number of either sensed or paced or combination events. In the Biotronik units, post-shock pacing can be programmed at separate higher value and also for a specified, programmable period of time, the Post Shock Duration, 30seconds to 30 minutes.

The other main reason for having post-shock pacing programmed separately is tissue refractoriness after the shock. Failure to capture is frequently noted after an ICD shock (Figure 5-16) and for that reason, it is recommended to program pacing output higher than the regular brady pacing parameter.

Post-shock pacing parameters are programmable separately for reasons that are specific to post shock situation, such as increased risk for arrhythmia and tissue refractoriness

---

- Bradycardia pacing consists of basic bradycardia support and post-shock pacing. Basic bradycardia pacing can be programmed similar to typical pacemaker programming. Post-shock pacing should be programmed with some delay and lower rate to avoid re-induction of VT, as well as at a higher output to overcome tissue refractoriness.
- The rates for bradycardia support is, in most ICDs, limited by the lowest VT zone (ELA Defender allows for some overlap).
- Bradycardia basic (e.g. refractory periods) and advance features (e.g. mode switch, rate smoothing, rate stabilization) can be programmed based on clinical setting.

Follow up Care

General Considerations

The follow up care of ICD patients differs from pacemaker in several aspects. The most significant difference lies in the fundamental principle of the indication for the device. The patient with ICD has suffered or is considered to be at risk for sudden death. Thus, at least, there is a concern for increased mortality, even if the device itself is intended to reduce such a risk. In addition, the patient with ICD generally has an underlying heart disease and is therefore at risk for other cardiac morbidity. Another principle difference is the device mode of operation. The ICD operates by delivering a high-energy shock to terminate arrhythmia. The anticipation and real reaction to it is significantly more pronounced than the most bothersome discomfort from a pacemaker therapy. And unlike with the pacemaker, ICD therapy only occurs infrequently. Thus, up until the current models that are equipped with patient's alert modes, any small change in its operation may not give any warning and since the consequence of a malfunction of the device can be potentially fatal, there is a greater need for a "perfect" performance of the device.

The other significant difference between an ICD and a pacemaker is the fact that the ICD has more components to its hardware and software. In the past, this would mean a much larger device with a very short longevity and the patient would have had to undergo a much more extensive surgical procedure that carries a significant rate of post-operative morbidity. Nowadays, the surgical approach is much simpler and, in principle, is very similar to a pacemaker implantation. However, the total device system would still require slightly larger pulse generator and lead(s) and its operation is more complex.

The General Goals of ICD Follow Up:

1.	Monitoring ICD generator and lead performance
2.	Optimizing programming of tachyarrhythmia detection and therapy
3.	Optimizing programming of bradycardia support to tailor to clinical demand without negatively affecting tachyarrhythmia parameters
4.	Maximizing ICD pulse-generator longevity and anticipating the need for replacement accurately
5.	Addressing any need for concomitant antiarrhythmic drug therapy
6.	Addressing any need for supportive physical, psychological, and social care

Personnel and Equipment

The follow up facility must have the appropriate personnel and equipment. The personnel should consist of a physician who is experienced in all aspects of ICD performance and arrhythmia management, an experienced cardiovascular nurse, and technical support staff. A cardiovascular nurse who is also experienced in device programming can also function as the technical support personnel but technical assistance should at least be available through telephone contact. The equipment should consist of the appropriate programmer, an ECG recorder or monitor, and an emergency crash cart with an external defibrillator. For evaluation of older ICD models, a doughnut magnet would also be necessary.

For extended evaluation of ICD and overall management of the patient's arrhythmia, other facilities may be needed, such as an ambulatory electrocardiography laboratory that is equipped with several choices of monitoring such as 24-hour Holter and event recorders, exercise stress test laboratory, and radiologic and echocardiographic imaging facilities.

Follow up Frequency

There is no general consensus on what would be considered the most appropriate frequency for ICD follow up. At the beginning, immediately after its implantation, ICD should be followed up at intervals that would be appropriate for the evaluation of surgical healing and lead stability. In general, an outpatient visit at one week, one month, and three months would suffice. Afterwards, "routine" evaluation frequency is mainly dictated by the need for capacitor formation or reformation (Chapter 4). The appropriate frequency for capacitor formation is not uniform. Infrequent reformation would result in prolongation in the ICD charge time; however, too frequent reformation would result in earlier battery depletion and shorter device longevity. In weighing these opposing factors, capacitor reformation is best performed every three to six months. For this reason, it is customary to have the patient come for capacitor maintenance and other follow up evaluation at every three to six months.

Automatic capacitor reformation that is now available in most ICD models is also performed at every three or six month interval. CPI units re-form the capacitors every three months, Medtronic every six months, Ventritex programmable (recommended every three to six months), ELA every six months, and Biotronik every four months. With this feature, the patient does not need to come to clinic for manual capacitor maintenance, but a visit would still be necessary for evaluating the outcome of the automatic performance.

In addition to the "routine" visit, the patient may need to be seen for other antiarrhythmic management as well as overall cardiovascular evaluation. Such a need ranges from minimal, such as in patients with minimal structural heart disease) to significant, such as in patients with frequent ICD therapy requiring adjustment of their antiarrhythmic drug regimen.

> **Follow-up frequency is based on general clinical need as current devices are now equipped with automatic capacitor reformation**

Routine Analysis of ICD

The maintenance of ICD operation includes the assessment of the unit's functions and lead(s) integrity. At each regular visit, the ICD must be interrogated for the assessment of, at least, device status, programmed parameters and therapy history. Lead(s) integrity assessment usually requires sensing and pacing threshold measurement and, sometimes, high-energy shock delivery. Accessing each item requires familiarity with the specific programmer.

Familiarity with a certain brand is helpful as the information obtain from interrogation of its devices are usually formatted similarly for that same brand. Otherwise, the clinician must go through the long list of the data shown and printed. Due to the significant amount of information now contained within each device and during its interrogation, not all of the data would be available on a single screen. Hence the clinician must also be familiar with the sub-screens and how to access them. Examples of basic interrogation are shown below.

```
 Episode Counters
                                  Since Last        Device
                                    Cleared          Totals
                                  14-MAR-00
 Treated
   VF Therapy                         0                 3
   VT Therapy                         0                 1
   VT-1 Therapy                       0                 3
   Commanded Therapy                  0                 1
 Nontreated
   No Therapy Programmed              0                 0
   Nonsustained Episodes            70               259
 Total Episodes                     70               267
```

```
 Device Parameter Summary     Tachy Mode =      Monitor+Therapy

 VF    200 bpm                                  17J/ 31J/ 31J X 3
       1.0 sec

 VT    170 bpm    Onset = OFF         ATP1x  3  14J/ 31J/ 31J X 3
       5.0 sec    Stab Inhibit = 40 ms ATP2x OFF
                  Stab Shock = OFF
                  SRD = 3:00 min:sec
                              BRADY         POST-SHOCK
 Mode                         VVIR          VVI
 Lower Rate Limit              60  ppm       60  ppm
 Max Sensor Rate              120  ppm       --  ppm
 Vent Ampl and Pulse Width    5.0 V,  0.5 ms 7.5 V,  1.0 ms
 Enable Magnet Use                                ON
   Change Tachy Mode with Magnet                  ON
 Beep During Capacitor Charge                     OFF
 Beep on Sensed V Events and Paced V Events       OFF
 Beep when ERI is Reached                         ON
 Electrogram Storage
   Ventricular                                    ON
   Shock                                          ON
 EGM Onset Storage                                ON
```

```
 AICD Device Data

 Last Interrogation                    02-JUN-00 10:04
 Last Re-programming                   23-MAR-00 13:14
 Last Delivered Shock                  10-MAR-00 18:48
   Energy                                    14 J
   Charge Time                              0.4 sec
   Shocking Impedance                        38 Ω
 Auto Capacitor Re-form                      90 days
 Last Capacitor Re-form                23-APR-00 13:56
   Charge Time                              8.8 sec
 Cumulative Charge Time                01:17 min:sec
 Battery Status                             BOL
   Monitoring Voltage                      6.43 V
   Charging Voltage                        5.06 V
 Implant Duration                             5 months
```

```
 Lead System Data

                     Implant Date   Previous      This
                     24-JAN-00      Results       Follow-up
 Ventricular
 R-Wave Ampl         N/R mV         18.53 mV      16.91 mV
 Impedance           N/R Ω           1065 Ω         1041 Ω
 Ampl Threshold      N/R           0.4V @  0.5ms  0.4V @  0.5ms
 PW Threshold        N/R            N/R           N/R
```

All energies reported as stored.

Figure 5-12. This is an example of a printout of basic interrogation of a CPI unit. It consists of episode counters, programmed parameters, device status, and lead status. This is the minimal amount of information needed.

Mar 03, 2000 12:09:53
9962 Software Version 2.0
Copyright (c) Medtronic, Inc. 1997

ICD Model: Gem 7227
Serial Number: PIP101645H

Status Report   Page 1

Last Interrogation: Mar 03, 2000 12:00:21

Battery Voltage

(ERI=2.55 V, EOL=2.40 V)

Mar 03, 2000 12:00:15
Voltage   2.97 V

Last Capacitor Formation*

Oct 24, 1999 04:45:40
Charge Time   10.08 sec
Energy   0.0 - 35.0 J

Last Charge

Nov 22, 1999 17:52:50
Charge Time   2.85 sec
Energy   0.1 - 15.0 J

*Minimum Auto Cap Formation Interval is 6 months.

Lead Impedance

Mar 03, 2000 03:00:04
V. Pacing   410 ohms
Defibrillation (HVB)   17 ohms

Last High Voltage Therapy

Nov 22, 1999 17:52:51
Measured Impedance   35 ohms
Delivered Energy   14.4 J
Waveform   Biphasic
Pathway   B>AX

Device Status

Charge Circuit is OK.

Mar 03, 2000 12:10:03
9962 Software Version 2.0
Copyright (c) Medtronic, Inc. 1997

ICD Model: Gem 7227
Serial Number: PIP101645H

Quick Look Report   Page 1

Last Interrogation: Mar 03, 2000 12:00:21
Episodes Last Interrogated: Mar 03, 2000 12:00:21

Since Last Session: Nov 22, 1999

Episodes

VF   0
FVT   0
VT   1
SVT/NST   11

% Pacing

Sensed   5 %
Paced   94 %

Current Data

Battery Voltage

(ERI=2.55 V, EOL=2.40 V)
Mar 03, 2000   2.97 V

Last Full Energy Charge

Oct 24, 1999   10.08 sec

Last Capacitor Formation

Oct 24, 1999

Lead Impedance

Mar 03, 2000
V. Pacing   410 ohms
Defibrillation (HVB)   17 ohms

Figure 5-13. Shown above are two pages of the printout of an interrogation of a Medtronic GEM 7227 unit. The top page, Status Report, shows device status. The lower page, Quick Look is the first page of a summary of the basic interrogation containing episode counters, brief device status, and programmed parameters (not shown here).

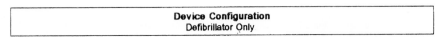

Device Configuration
Defibrillator Only

Detection Criteria		Tachyarrhythmia Therapies	
Fib Detection: 330 ms (182 bpm)		Fib Therapy:	[1] 695 V
			[2] 800 V
			[3] 800 V x 4
		Waveform:	Biphasic
			+ 4.0 ms, - 3.5 ms
			RV Polarity: Anode (+)
Morphology Scoring: Off			
Bradycardia Pacing			
Pacing: VVI 50 ppm Hysteresis: Off			
Brady Output: 5.0 V, 0.5 ms			
Refractory Period: 375 ms			
Post-therapy Pause: 1 sec			

Capacitor Maintenance	
Maintenance Interval: 3 months	Maintenance Voltage: 800 V

Electrogram Storage Parameters	
Number (Duration) of stored events: 29 Events (32 sec)	Duration of Pre-Trigger: 28 sec
Event Trigger: Sinus	Resolution: Nominal
EGM Source: Bipole	
Events Stored: Fib	

Real-Time Measurements	
Unloaded Battery Voltage: >3.2 V	Auto Gain Setting: 0
Pacing Lead Impedance: 640 ohms	R-Wave Amplitude: >9 mV

Figure 5-14. Shown above is the first page of an interrogation of a St.Jude/Ventritex unit. This usually contains programmed parameters and device status. Therapy history (not shown) is available on subsequent pages.

Device Status Evaluation

In reviewing device status, it is important to assess the battery status and the result of the last capacitor re-formation. Near the end of battery's life, the battery voltage would be low and the "charge time" during capacitor re-formation would be longer. By assessing the voltage of the battery and its trend, the remainder of the battery's life can be estimated.

For a single-battery ICD, the battery voltage would go from approximately 3.1-3.2 volts at its beginning of life (BOL) and drop to about 2.5 volts at the end of life/service (EOL/EOS) (Figure 5-15). At around 2.55 volts, the battery would have about one to three months of normal operation and this status is used as an indicator for elective replacement (ERI). With a two-battery ICD, the voltages would be approximately 6.1-6.2 V at BOL and 4.4-4.5 V at EOL/EOS with ERI usually set at 4.9-5.1 V.

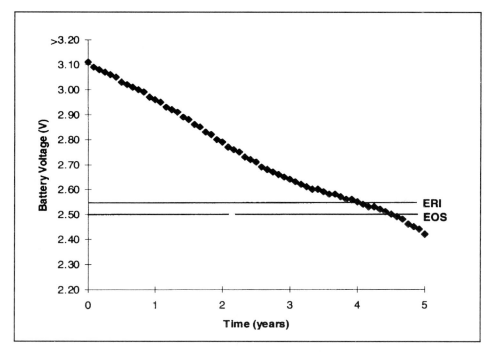

Figure 5-15. A typical decline of a single battery voltage, starting from 3.1-3.2 V at BOL to 2.4-2.5 V at EOL/EOS in a St.Jude/Ventritex unit. Just prior to reaching EOL/EOS, the generator should be replaced electively (ERI) (Reproduced withpermission from St.Jude).

The capacitor charge/charging time depends on the battery status and hence, it provides additional information of ICD longevity. In estimating battery's life from the charge time, it should be noted that the charge time also depends on whether it is a single or double battery ICD. Charge times for single-battery ICD would typically be twice as long as those of a double-battery unit. Typically, a double-battery ICD would need 6-7 seconds to fully charge to 30 joules, while a single-battery unit would need 12-13 seconds. When the battery reaches ERI, the charge time would come close to 10 seconds for a double-battery ICD and 20 seconds for a single-battery unit.

Assessing Programmed Parameters

The first step in reviewing programmed parameters, is to confirm that all entries are the same as at the previous visit. The ICD, like pacemakers, is susceptible to electromagnetic interference (see Interaction with Electromagnetic Source section). High frequency signals from electromagnetic interference can cause reprogramming of the ICD through the "noise response" or "noise reversion" mode. Such interference would cause oversensing in both bradycardia and tachycardia detection modes, thus it would cause "noise response" (which is programmable to various modes) and trigger therapy for tachycardia. In some devices, the noise reversion mode also operates in the tachycardia detection scheme and therefore, therapy could be inhibited.

Although rare, there are still occurrences of accidental reprogramming due to exposure to a strong magnetic field. In some ICD units (CPI), exposure to magnet for >30 seconds can turn off the unit's tachyarrhythmia (detection and therapy) operation (see below). In others, the units would be "blinded" only for the period of time that it is exposed to the magnet.

Reviewing Therapy History

The therapy history is the part that the patient is most interested in. The result of this interrogation frequently triggers a mixed reaction. If an episode of tachyarrhythmia were detected, it would frequently trigger some degree of fear (that the occurrence of a high-energy shock might be imminent soon). However, if no arrhythmia or therapy were detected at all after long term follow up, it would raise the question whether the ICD would have been needed at all.

The content of therapy history is usually very straightforward and self-explanatory. However, it should be noted that the ICD interpretation of the tachyarrhythmia should be confirmed, especially the classification of the arrhythmia into non-tachycardia, VT, or VF, because such classification is purely based on the programmed criteria. In the earlier models, when only no or few parameter (R-R) intervals was available, it would be very difficult to confirm the accuracy of the ICD interpretation of the event. Now, with the availability of local and far-field EGM, the retrieved data provide more clinical information. With the availability of dual-chamber information, both the ICD and the physician can make even more precise interpretation.

Data from therapy history can be used to fine tune tachyarrhythmia detection and therapy. Appropriateness and accuracy of detection enhancements such as Onset, Stability, EGM Width, or Morphology, can be assessed. Therapy can also be changed if necessary, such as increasing or decreasing the number of ATP attempts or adding or eliminating low-energy cardioversion. Finally, the frequency and severity of VT or VF episode should be taken into the patient's overall clinical situation with specific attention paid to antiarrhythmic drug regimen.

In this context, the presence and frequency of atrial arrhythmias should also be noted. Since most ICD units are not equipped with atrial antitachycardia pacing or defibrillation, the management of atrial arrhythmia must be dealt with antiarrhythmic drug. However, appropriateness of SVT discrimination, double tachycardia detection, and mode switch features should be scrutinized.

Assessing Lead(s) Integrity

Assessment of ICD lead(s) function and integrity includes the measurements of pace/sense and high-voltage lead parameters. The evaluation of pace/sense lead consists of measuring sensing and pacing thresholds and impedance, much in the same way as the assessment of pacemaker leads. In contrast, the high-voltage lead can not be assessed with such methods. To completely assure its adequate performance, defibrillation capacity, and impedance must be tested. Obviously, in most cases, this would not be practical and therefore, data are only collected from the most recent delivered therapy. Thus, in the first few months after implantation, if no spontaneous event with therapy have occurred, it is customary to perform an elective VF induction for the assessment of sensing and defibrillation adequacy. Afterwards, it is assumed that the chronic lead would remain stable in terms of its anatomic location and electrical properties. It is, however, evident that deterioration in high-voltage lead can escape detection and be discovered only at operative testing during generator replacement. For this reason, it is argued that DFT testing should be regularly performed such as at yearly interval.

In the latest models from Medtronic (GEM) and CPI (Prizm), the high-voltage lead integrity can be assessed by delivering a subthreshold pulse, which would enable the measurement of impedance at that pulse strength.

In addition to assessment of device status, pacing and sensing stability, and lead integrity, routine analysis of ICD must include careful review of therapy history and the device interpretation of the arrhythmia must be confirmed by the clinician by interpreting the electrogram

---

- Routine outpatient analysis of ICD should at least include assessment of device and lead (if available) status, programmed parameters, and episode counters.
- Device status data would provide information on battery and capacitor status and device longevity. Lead status would give information on lead integrity and any trend or changes in pacing, sensing and impedance parameters.
- Programmed parameters should be reviewed to assess its appropriateness for clinical status and if there have been any (deliberate or inadvertent) changes.
- Episode counter, which is usually the information that the patient would be most interested in, provides patient's clinical progress in terms of arrhythmia recurrence. Any episode that is significant is now kept in the device's memory and should be analyzed carefully. If available, EGM for each episode should be analyzed to confirm appropriateness of detection and therapy.
- Analysis of pacing history, if available, should also be analyzed for appropriateness of sensing, tracking, and mode-switching.
- Sensing and pacing threshold should be done periodically.

Some Practical Steps in ICD Management

The ICD Response to Magnet Application

Magnet application, if used properly, can be helpful with ICD as it is with pacemaker. However, the ICD response to magnet is quite different. Magnet primarily affects the tachyarrhythmia operation of the unit, which is quite helpful in emergency situation where therapy (such as shocks) needs to be aborted. Its most frequent application is in the Operating Room, when a programmer may not be accessible.

With most ICD units, magnet application would simply inhibit tachyarrhythmia detection and therapy ("blind" the ICD) during the time that the magnet is in close proximity to the unit. However, the CPI unit has several programmable magnet response features. First of all, the ICD can be programmed to either respond or not respond to magnet application. If the "Enable Magnet Use" feature is turned ON, the ICD could perform the magnet functions. There are three magnet functions. One is to emit an audible tone to indicate whether the units "tachy" mode is active (R-wave tracking tone) or inactive (continuous tone). The second is to inhibit tachyarrhythmia therapy and induction ("blinding" function). The third is to allow for programming the "Change Tachy Mode With Magnet" function. Then the "Change Tachy Mode With Magnet" function can be programmed to ON (to allow a change the unit's tachyarrhythmia mode with > 30-second magnet application) or OFF.

The effect of magnet on bradycardia parameters varies among the different manufacturers, but commonly these parameters would not be affected at all (CPI, Medtronic, Ventritex, and Biotronik). In some ICD units (ELA), magnet application would affect bradycardia pacing by reprogramming it to the "magnet rate" which can be used as the battery's life indicator (94 or 96 bpm at BOL, 80 bpm at ERI, and 77 bpm at EOL) at maximum amplitude (voltage and pulse width).

ICD response to magnet is most useful under emergency situation. In the event of multiple inappropriate shock, magnet can be applied by medical staff (paramedics, Emergency Room staff, or Clinic staff) once the patient has been placed on monitor. The unit will be immediately "blinded" and no longer able to detect. Such maneuver is also useful in the Operating Room when electrocautery is used while the device has not been deactivated.

For concern of inappropriate usage, magnets are usually not supplied to the patient. However, if potential device malfunction is suspected or if there is a history of frequent inappropriate shocks from atrial fibrillation which can not be averted by reprogramming, a magnet can be provided to the patient for emergency use but the patient should be advised to use it only after the arrival of medical personnel, such as the paramedics.

Radiographic Identification

In the not so rare instances that information of ICD model could not be obtained from history, the manufacturer identification can be retrieved from the generator radiographic image. Typically the logo, or at times the actual unit model inscription is radio-opaque (Figure 5-16).

This information can be crucial, especially if interrogation is necessary to assess patient's symptom and his/her clinical progress.

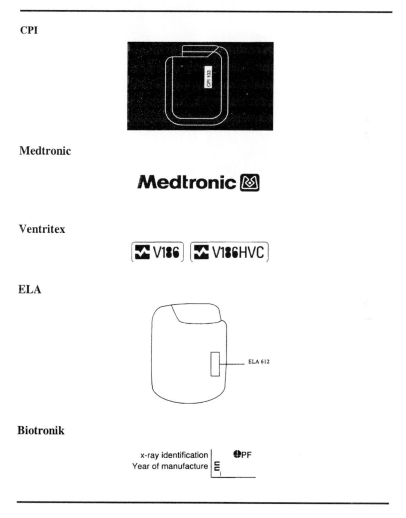

Figure 5-16. Radiographic identification of the various manufacturers (Reproduced with permission from the respective manufacturers).

It would also be useful to become familiar with the typical radiographic image of certain ICD lead system because of the various types of leads. For example, the SVC coil lead with the early Medtronic units is a separate lead "hanging" near the SVC can be mistaken for a dislodged atrial lead.

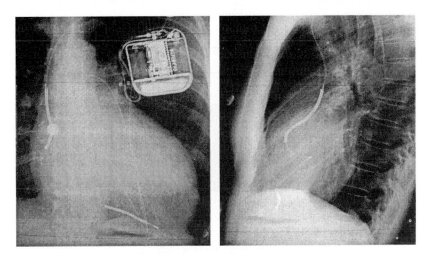

Figure 5-17. Shown above are PA and lateral chest X-ray views of an RV endocardial lead with dual coil. The proximal coil typically resides within the SVC area.

The presence of two coils within a single right ventricular lead (Figure 5-17) can also be confusing to the radiologist.

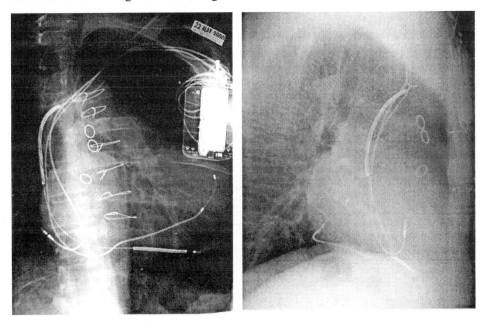

Figure 5-18. Shown above is a biventricular system with the LV lead in the midcardiac vein

Lately, with the increasing use of bi-ventricular lead, the coronary sinus lead can be mistaken as dislodged or misplaced pacemaker lead. The position of the left ventricular lead in a biventricular pacing/ICD system can be quite variable (see also Chapter 6). The most common location is within the posterolateral branch of the coronary sinus, but other locations are also used, such as the midcardiac vein (Figure 5-18).

- Application of a large (donut shape) magnet will "blind" the ICD such that detection is non-operational. This can be quite helpful in an emergency setting when immediate deactivation of the ICD is necessary, such as in the event of incessant, multiple shocks due to inappropriate detection of sinus tachycardia, atrial fibrillation or noise. It can also be helpful during surgery when electrocautery usage is needed and the ICD has not been deactivated.
- Chest radiography can be helpful in identifying the brand of an ICD if the information can not be obtained otherwise.
- Chest radiography of ICD can be confusing to the radiologist because of the variety of ICD leads and defibrillation coils. It is even more confusing nowadays with the use of additional leads for biventricular pacing.

Interactions with Drugs and Pacemakers

Interaction with Antiarrhythmic Drugs

Although antiarrhythmic drugs are not commonly used as the primary therapy for the management of VT/VF, they are frequently used as concomitant treatment. The common practice in utilizing drugs is to prescribe them after the implantation of ICD and typically, after the occurrence of frequent shocks. With the addition of antiarrhythmic drug, it is hoped that frequency of VT/VF may be reduced and that the VT may become slower and more responsive to ATP. It should be kept in mind that even if such goals for improving the patient's quality of life can be achieved, the drug may also affect the operation of ICD adversely.

Effects of Antiarrhythmic Drugs on Defibrillation Threshold

Antiarrhythmic drugs may alter the DFT by various mechanisms including their effect on repolarization and transmembrane potential. In general, drugs with sodium-channel blocking properties tend to raise the DFT while those with potassium-channel blockade tend to lower it, probably through extension of repolarization.[61-63]   Thus, pure Vaughan-Williams class I drugs such as flecainide and encainide increase the DFT while class III drugs such as sotalol and many newer members of the class lower it.[62-70]   Those with mixed properties such as quinidine, procainamide and disopyramide, interestingly, have no significant effect on the DFT.[6,71-73]   Of note, acute administration of procainamide, without its metabolite effect, increases DFT as expected.[74]

Table 5-1. The Effects of Antiarrhythmic Drugs on DFT

Increase	No Change	Decrease
Amiodarone (chronic)		Amiodarone (acute)
Propafenone	Propafenone	Propafenone (acute)
Flecainide (chronic)		
Flecainide (acute)	Flecainide (acute)	
Encainide	MODE	
(ODE)		
Procainamide (acute)	Procainamide (chronic)	NAPA
	Quinidine	
	Disopyramide	
Lidocaine (acute)	Mexiletine (acute & chronic)	
		Sotalol (acute & chronic)
		Ibutilide (acute)
		Azimilide (acute)
		Tedisamil (acute)

Amiodarone, which also has mixed properties, however, is well known for raising the DFT, even to significantly higher values.[4,75-78]   Thus, the DFT can also be affected through are other factors that are yet to be explained.   In some experiments, some drugs that are known to increase DFT have no effects when given intravenously[79] or have different effects in different animal species.[79,80] In fact, intravenous amiodarone and propafenone were noted to lower DFT.[81] Lidocaine increases DFT while its congener mexiletine does not affect it in most reports.[74,82-84]   However, both drugs, when added to flecainide, were noted to cause incremental increase in DFT [85].   It has also been reported that the effect of antiarrhythmic drug on DFT is dependent on defibrillation electrode and waveform system.

For example, the effects were noted to be less with the use of biphasic waveform. Table 5-1 lists the known, general effect of antiarrhythmic drugs on DFT.

Effects of Antiarrhythmic Drugs on Arrhythmia Detection

The electrophysiologic influence of antiarrhythmic drug on tachyarrhythmia can cause beneficial and deleterious effects on ICD operation. The major purpose of antiarrhythmic drug use is to slow the VT as to become more responsive to ATP. While this may very well be the outcome, other effects should be anticipated. The same mechanism that operates on the drug effect on the rate of VT may increase the frequency of arrhythmia and make the arrhythmia incessant. The drug can also produce electrophysiological changes to the baseline rhythm that may affect the device's operation, such as significant slowing of sinus rate and significant increases in PR segment, QRS duration and QT interval. Significant sinus bradycardia and chronotropic incompetence can cause pacemaker syndrome in patients with single-chamber ICD. Significant PR-segment prolongation can cause an increase in AV pacing and, possibly, unnecessary ventricular dysynchronous contraction leading to worsening heart failure. A significant increase in QRS duration may cause potential double counting and similarly, excessive QT prolongation may cause T-wave oversensing. These potential problems, however, can be easily prevented with careful scrutiny and clinical follow up.

> **Antiarrhythmic drugs can affect the patient with an ICD several ways and in some instance the adverse effects, such as those on the DFT and VT rate can be detrimental**

Interaction with Pacemakers

Obviously, with the use of ICD with pacemaker properties, interaction with pacemaker is no longer a major issue. In the past, a separate pacemaker is frequently needed because the simple VVI pacemaker within the ICD would not be sufficient. Typically, a separate pacemaker unit would be needed to provide dual-chamber support or rate responsive mode.

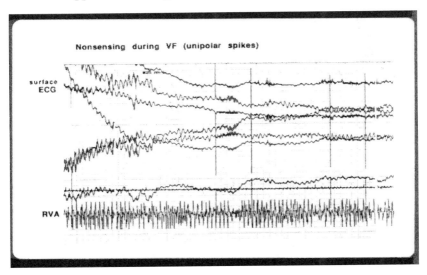

Figure 5-19. This tracing was recorded during DFT testing where VF was not sensed by the pacemaker, which in turns, deliver pacing output that interfered with VF detection and resulted in prolonged VF episode.

The pacemaker may become a source of external stimulus that could interfere with the ICD detection scheme. Of common occurrence is the double or multiple counting that would then result into false tachyarrhythmia detection. Of even more serious consequence is the interference with VF detection. In the worst scenario where the pacemaker fails to recognized VF and delivers pacing output, the ICD sensing gain control would be reset to a lower sensitivity level by these stimulus artifact and would not be able to adjust fast enough to detect the underlying small signals from VF. Such a scenario is more likely to occur with the use of pacemaker with unipolar pacing output (Figure 5-19). For those reasons, unipolar pacemaker is contraindicated in patients with an ICD.

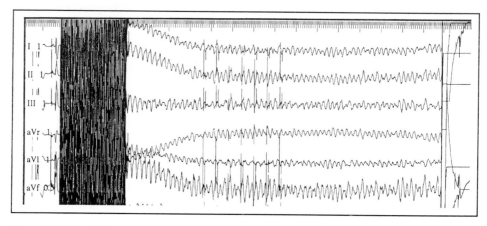

Figure 5-20A. This tracing was recorded during testing of ICD-Pacemaker interaction. The patient, who only recently received a new CPI MINI generator was noted to require brady pacing support for chronotropic incompetence. Thus, a separate DDDR pacemaker with a dedicated bipolar mode was implanted. The two steps of assessment were performed. First, it was assessed whether the VF was appropriately sensed by the pacemaker and resulted in appropriate inhibition. Then a magnet was applied over the pacemaker to produce a DOO mode and the ICD assessed for possible pacemaker output sensing and interference with the automatic gain control (Figure 5-20B)

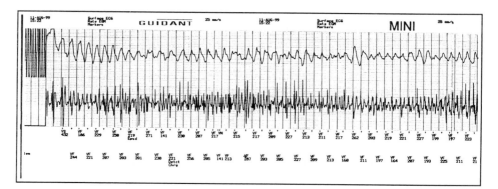

Figure 5-20B. The tracing shows a recording of the same episode of Figure 5-20A, with surface ECG lead V6 and local integrated bipolar EGM. The EGM of the ICD did not register any sensing of pacing output. There was no pacing output noted on the EGM despite the apparent large "spikes" on the surface ECG in Figure 5-15A. The absence of such interference is important to assess.

If a separate pacemaker is to be implanted along with an ICD, only a "dedicated" bipolar unit (a pacemaker that would not "revert" to unipolar after a shock) should be used and the possibility for negative ICD-pacemaker interactions must be assessed. This is best performed in the laboratory during VF induction. The first step is to assess the sensing capability of the pacemaker during VF. Then, the pacemaker should be programmed to asynchronous mode (by applying a magnet) with maximum output to assess the ability of the ICD to detect VF during the pacemaker output interference (Figure 5-20). In our experience, bipolar pacemaker output rarely interferes with ICD recognition of VT or VF.

Another potential negative interaction involves the ICD influence on the pacemaker. Theoretically, the high-energy shock from the ICD can cause noise reversion or even permanent damage to the pacemaker, similar to reprogramming and damage that are caused by external shocks. Such incidence, however, has not been reported to occur.

Finally, the separate pacemaker is not equipped to anticipate tissue refractoriness to pacing after a high-energy shock. Thus, the programmed bradycardia output parameters may have to be tested for appropriateness during the post-shock time period. If the output is programmed to a value based on routine bradycardia status, failure to capture maybe observed after an ICD shock.

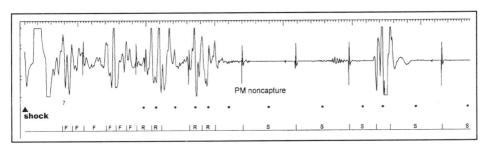

Figure 5-21. This tracing was recorded from an episode of a prolonged VF due to interference from a separate PM. After the shock, when VF ceased, the output from the pacemaker was not sufficient to capture the more refractory tissue. This example underscores the need for programming post shock pacing at higher output, which would not be an available feature with a separate pacemaker unit.

> **Potential negative interaction between the ICD and a separate pacemaker should be addressed, including VF non-sensing by the pacemaker, pacing stimulus over-sensing by the ICD, and post-shock pacing problems**

Interactions with Electromagnetic Field

Electromagnetic interference (EMI) may cause false detection or noise response resulting in inappropriate therapy or inhibition of appropriate therapy. In more serious circumstances, the EMI can cause permanent damage to the generator. Many hospital equipment involve electromagnetic field and the physician should be familiar with the potential of such negative interaction.

One such equipment is electrocautery, which uses radiofrequency current to cut or coagulate tissue.[86,87] To a pacemaker, it would be interpreted as noise and automatic reprogramming to a noise reversion mode would result. To the ICD, such high frequency signal could cause false tachyarrhythmia sensing and inappropriate therapy. Such a mishap, electrocautery should be used in short bursts. It is recommended that the tachyarrhythmia detection be deactivated during any surgery involving electrocautery. In general, the closer the electrocautery unit is to the ICD and its lead(s)system, the more likely interference would occur.[86] After the surgery, the parameters of the ICD should be interrogated. Similarly, tachyarrhythmia detection should be deactivated during an ablation using radiofrequency energy and all parameters interrogated after completion of the procedure.[88] External defibrillation and cardioversion can cause damage to the ICD generator if placed closed (< 6 inches) to the unit.

The use of MRI can cause more serious damage to an ICD or a pacemaker. The strong electromagnetic field can cause noise detection as well as rapid pacing.[89] In addition, the strong magnetic field can cause movements of the iron-containing pulse generator and permanent damage to it.

Lithotripsy also generates high-energy vibration and can cause noise detection resulting in pacemaker inhibition and/or tachyarrhythmia detection.[90] Hence it is also recommended that tachyarrhythmia detection be deactivated during such therapy. Similar risk can also occur with diathermy, but the effect is less if it is applied away from the unit. Transcutaneous electric nerve stimulation (TENS) units, which puts out high-frequency stimulation, can also cause interference but if placed at a distance away from the ICD or leads, its effect may not be significant.[91] To be sure, it may be wise to test the effect of the TENS unit on the ICD detection. Dental drilling does not cause noise production to a pacemaker or ICD. Dental ultrasound scaling, although potentially can cause electrical noise, does not seem to be harmful to pacemaker function either. Radiation therapy does not cause signal interference but it can cause damage to the semi-conductor materials.[92]

Strong electromagnetic field is also common in industrial environment. Thus the patient is advised to avoid such area. For example, the patient with ICD is generally advised against using arc welding. However, the actual strength of EMI and its effect on the ICD can be tested if such exposure can not be reasonably assured. In this era of increasing number and types of electromagnetic equipment, patients are concerned of the possibility of an adverse effect from general day to day environment. Of the common sources of EMI in public area are pagers, cellular telephones and electronic surveillance devices.

Data from several studies assessing the effects of cellular telephone indicate that adverse effects from these devices do occur but rarely. In general, the stronger the EMI source and the closer the source is to the ICD, the more likely the occurrence of negative interactions. With respect to cellular telephone, car phones are significantly stronger than hand-held ones, but hand-held units are typically placed closer to the body. It is thus advised that a hand-held cellular phone be placed at least 6 inches away from the ICD. In the case of pectoral ICD, it would be more practical to simply use the phone on the opposite ear.[93] It was noted that digital phones have greater potential for EMI interference and that unipolar devices are more susceptible.[94] Transmission from cellular telephone tower antenna does not seem to affect devices.[95]

The effects of electronic article surveillance (EAS) systems have also been tested.[96-100] In all of the studies performed, some effects were noted but only when exposure was prolonged and close to the device. Abdominally placed devices and older models seem to be more susceptible. It is recommended, therefore, that patients go through these surveillance systems in a normal walking pace and not to come too close in contact with them.

It is of interest to see the data of some studies showing the safety of using arc welding and bipolar electrocautery equipment in ICD patients.[101,102]

Electromagnetic field can affect ICD as it does pacemaker, thus the patient is advised to avoid such presence including common household equipment such as portable cellular telephones

---

- Antiarrhythmic drugs can be clinically useful for the ICD patient but can affect significant effects on device operation. Most Na^+-channel blockers increase DFT while K^+-channel blockers typically lowers DFT. Amiodarone is known to raise DFT significantly. Antiarrhythmic drugs can also affect VT rate significantly and therefore, detection parameters should be reassessed
- If a separate pacemaker unit is present, interaction between the two devices should be assessed. Pacemaker output, if not inhibited, during VF can affect detection. Therefore unipolar pacemaker is contraindicated in the ICD patient. The function of separate pacemaker may also be altered by ICD shock and furthermore, post-shock tissue refractoriness may cause non-capture.
- Electromagnetic field can significantly affect ICD operation. Thus the use of some equipment (such as MRI) is contraindicated. Other equipment with electrical or electromagnetic output can be used with caution. It would be advisable to test their usage (e.g. diathermy, TENS units) and if possible, the ICD should be activated (e.g. with electrocautery, lithotripsy). Common household equipment can be used with caution (i.e. by maintaining some distance).

Quality of Life Aspects

In addition to the ICD beneficial effects on mortality and morbidity, the quality of life aspects of the device therapy are important to the patients. The quality of life is generally assessed on the basis of four conditions: physical, psychological, social, and everyday activities.[103]

Quality of life in ICD patients has been addressed in several studies.[9,14,104-107] In one study[106], a significant number of patients suffered from reduced quality of life. Of the many concerns, the most common issues revolve aroung physical appearance and limitation (such as activity and sex) and anxietyover receiving shocks. Most other studies, however, showed that despite initial fear and depression with respect to physical and social limitation from the device, most patients indicate improvement in overall quality of life after ICD implantation. In the Bonn study[9], most patients perceived improvement of quality of life.

A study reviewing the literature on the quality of life of ICD patients[9,14,104,108-110] also showed that patient's acceptance are generally good and that they would recommend it to others. Most patients returned to work but some refrained from driving, a major issue with ICD patients.[111-114] Fear and anxiety were the most common psychological issues, occurring between 24 to 85 % of ICD recipients, although clinically significant anxiety disorder ranges only from 13 to 34 %, which is similar to the incidence in other cardiovascular illnesses. Of importance is the observation that patients associate ICD shock with certain predisposing situation or behavior, similar to the experience with conditioning paradigm. This is especially true in younger patients.[108] Younger patients tend to socially isolate themselves, suffer sleep disturbances and limit their physical activity. Patients would need counseling to clarify this notion. Depression occurs in 24 to 33 % of patients, mostly caused by the feeling that they have no control over the occurrence of shock and those suffering greater than 5 shocks showed significant anxiety.[9]

Driving remains an important issue in ICD patients. There is yet a standard recommendation regarding driving limitations for patients with ICD. This is understandable from many point of views. ICD recipients are a diverse group of patients, many would rarely receive shock from their device. It is also not known how much future incidence of VT/VF and the therapy would affect driving performance. Furthermore, the incidence of driving accidents caused by ICD recipients is not known and is not likely to be significantly higher than patients who are at risk for VT/VF or syncope who do not have an ICD. Thus addressing driving limitations to ICD patients only would be perceived as unfair. Finally, driving privilege is almost essential for most people in the western world and limiting this privilege would severely handicap them socially and psychologically. Thus, there is a wide discrepancy in people and physician opinions regarding the recommendation for driving limitations.[115] Regardless of their physician recommendation, most ICD patients resume driving after 6 months.[116]

In outlining driving recommendation for ICD patients, it would be important to assess the clinical situation. In patients who survived a cardiac arrest, the highest recurrence rate is within the first one to three months[117] and this incidence decreases over the ensuing months. In patients who have not had a cardiac arrest, the likelihood for the first episode within the first year is low. It would also be important to assess the likelihood for syncope in individual patients[118] because not all patient would suffer serious hemodynamic consequences from the arrhythmia or its therapy. Obviously, the consequences of motor vehicle accident even in the rare likelihood of syncope must also be taken into consideration. Thus, commercial driving should probably be prohibited in all ICD recipients.

The European Study Group[119] outlines a proposal for driving recommendation based on the above considerations.

Table 5-2. Recommendations of the European Study Group

Patient Characteristics	Driving Recommendations
Prophylactic ICD patients	
VT/VF patients	
Commercial driving	Total restrictions
Non-commercial driving	Restriction for a defined period
Low recurrence rate	6-month driving-abstinence
Intermediate recurrence rate	Extended driving-abstinence*
High recurrence rate	Total restriction

* until reduction of recurrence rate or confirmation of absence of syncope

---

ICD therapy is live saving but it can affect the patient's quality of life such as physical limitations, employability, and driving privileges; hence these issues should be discussed and worked out

---

- ICD can affect quality of life, especially with physical activity and driving privileges. Support group may be beneficial.
- ICD shock and syncope during VT/VF may affect the person's cognitive function. The patient is advised to refrain from using heavy equipment or commercial driving. Regular driving privilege can be resumed in the absence of frequent syncope/VT/VF or ICD shock. Temporary abstinence is usually advised.

Trouble Shooting

Troubleshooting of the patient with an implantable cardioverter-defibrillator (ICD) requires a thorough understanding of basic ICD operation as well as sufficient knowledge of the specific functions of the unit in question. To familiarize with the specific features of all ICD units can be an overwhelming task as device's features are becoming increasingly complex and there is no uniformity among the various brands. Specific features of each of ICD models have been reviewed earlier. This section will outline the basic, common ICD problems with which the physician should be familiar and comfortable in managing.

Suspected Inappropriate Shocks

This is the most common complaint related to ICD therapy. A shock without an arrhythmia prodrome ("asymptomatic" shock) would typically frighten the patient and lead to a suspicion of device malfunction. The physician's initial role is to both reassure the patient of the appropriateness of his/her reaction and confirm that a shock in fact had been delivered. Most devices are now equipped with the time and date of a detected and treated arrhythmia and thus provide indisputable confirmation of the presence or absence of an "event". There have been reports of phantom shocks[120], which are likely due to an anxiety reaction to, perhaps, an overwhelming anticipation, which should be conveyed to the patient without putting blame. If a shock has indeed occurred, it should then be determined whether it was delivered (appropriately) for a tachyarrhythmia that had satisfied the programmed detection criteria or triggered by an abnormality in the sensing mechanism. It should be noted that inappropriate sensing does not necessarily indicate device malfunction.

Asymptomatic Tachyarrhythmia

Most devices can now provide detailed information on the event leading to the delivered therapy. Data on the R-R interval as well as the electrogram signal are usually available, providing useful information on the various characteristics of the arrhythmia. The dual-chamber ICDs, which provide data from atrial and ventricular channels, allow for greater accuracy in the diagnoses of the treated arrhythmia. It is not uncommon for the patient to not perceive symptoms from an arrhythmia[121,122] in spite of its apparent severity.

Ventricular tachycardia is typically detected by ICD within a few seconds and its therapy delivered soon afterwards. The time between the onset of VT and delivery of shock is typically short, about 10 seconds, especially with the newer devices; hence the arrhythmia can be nearly or completely asymptomatic. Although such rapid recognition and therapy delivery is potentially advantageous in preventing syncope and ensuring treatment efficacy, it provides the patient with very little warning. Thus, such patients would be typically startled by the unanticipated shock.

Another common scenario of an asymptomatic VT is encountered in the patient with a relatively slow, monomorphic VT. In such a patient, even a VT episode of a very long duration may not be perceived. Thus, even if shock therapy is delayed by several cycles of antitachycardia pacing, the patient may still be startled by the shock.

In either scenario, it would be helpful to inquire the patient about more subtle symptoms, such as mild lightheadedness, slight disorientation, diaphoresis, or vague chest discomfort. Obviously, the confirmation of VT can be readily obtained from interrogation of event EGM, which is now available in all newer generation ICDs.

Prior to the availability of "non-committed" therapy, it was common for patients to receive therapy for nonsustained VT (NSVT) because once an episode is detected, the device is committed to deliver the therapy. This is now a rare finding and if a shock is noted after the VT has self-terminated, the device should be interrogated to see if the non-committed feature had indeed been programmed. It should be noted that in some devices, confirmation of VT termination requires several consecutive long R-R intervals; hence in such instance, a non-committed therapy could still be delivered after the cessation of VT if there is insufficient time for such confirmation.

Although the rate and duration of VT provide useful information, it can not be assumed that a faster VT would cause more symptoms than a slower one. The clinical history with respect to the individual patient's tolerance to VT would be a better predictor to the amount of symptom that that patient would perceive prior to the ICD shock. Still, in many instances, the VT prior to shock would be considerably less symptomatic than the one at initial presentation because of the relatively rapid therapy delivery by the device.

Other tachyarrhythmias can be mistaken for VT by the device. Basic detection enhancement criteria such as sudden onset and stability are excellent in distinguishing sinus tachycardia and atrial fibrillation from VT[38,40,44,123-125] but may not adequately screen out paroxysmal supraventricular tachyarrhythmias or atrial flutter (AFL) with a regular 2:1 or 1:1 conduction. These arrhythmias would also have sudden onset and stable R-R intervals. More advanced detection enhancements may improve such screening, such as those involving atrial rhythm detection and local ventricular electrogram template.[47] But even with these detection enhancements, the ICD may still be unable to screen out supraventricular arrhythmias.[48,126] Identification of these arrhythmias would require a careful analysis of the event EGM. In the case of the patient who received shocks from atrial flutter or fibrillation, sometimes, the history alone is quite helpful. An episode of atrial flutter or fibrillation is frequently refractory to the ICD shock and thus, the patient would typically complaint of having received multiple repeated, consecutive shocks.

Sinus Tachycardia

Inappropriate therapy triggered by sinus tachycardia is a rare occurrence with current devices because the ICD detection can now be readily programmed to accommodate high exercise sinus rate and if necessary, enhancement criteria can be added. The few exceptions are the instances where there are significant overlaps between the slowest VT rate and the highest attainable sinus rate. In the very athletic patient, the peak exercise sinus rate may be well over 200 beats per minute and, hence, programming rate cut-off is problematic. While it would be desirable to program the rate cut-off above the maximum exercise heart rate, it might be risky to select a rate above 200/minute because VT can commonly occur at rates well below 200. Thus, discrimination between VT and sinus tachycardia may be difficult and typically the physician would choose to use a lower rate cut-off. In such instance, however, the absence of symptom prior to shock does not necessarily rule out VT, because the arrhythmia can be well tolerated hemodynamically. The event EGM would be helpful in identifying the nature of the arrhythmia. Then, an exercise stress test should be performed to assess the maximum sinus rate as well as to observe for cathecolamine-sensitive VT.

Oversensing

Oversensing is another common cause for asymptomatic shocks. In such a case, obviously, there is a complete absence of an arrhythmia symptom. Thus, if after a diligent history taking and careful analysis of the EGM an arrhythmia has been ruled out, the clinician should consider an oversensing problem.

Such a problem can be readily identified using the beep-o-gram method[127] or by observing simultaneous ECG and marker channels. Oversensing can be caused by various factors that do not necessarily represent a malfunction of the device, including the components of the intrinsic rhythm (T-wave, P-wave, or wide-QRS-complex oversensing) or by artificial pacemaker stimuli and other external stimuli.

T-wave or P-wave oversensing can occur, especially if the sensitivity setting is programmed very high. To ensure detection of fine VF, which can have a small R wave of 1 mV or less[128], it would be necessary, in most instances, to program sensitivity to the highest value. This, consequently, increases the likelihood for T-wave or P-wave oversensing. With devices utilizing an "auto gain control" (AGC), the sensitivity is automatically adjusted to the R wave and hence, in most cases where The R wave is adequate, there is a lower likelihood for T-wave or P-wave oversensing. Such oversensing possibility is usually scrutinized carefully during implantation. In any case, however, if a T-wave or P-wave oversensing is suspected, one should analyze the marker channel (or perform a beep-o-gram maneuver); then the possible causes for such delayed oversensing should be determined, such as changes in R-wave signal progressive myocardial deterioration or lead dislodgment.

T-wave oversensing can also be accentuated during sinus tachycardia (Figure 5-22). In such a case, even using discriminatory parameters such as onset criterion would not eliminate the problem because T-wave oversensing would start abruptly. Such a problem is also frequently frustrating because at baseline, T-wave oversensing is not present. With the availability of EGM within the therapy history greatly helps in identifying such a problem.

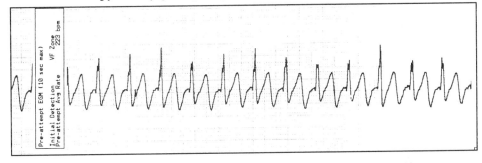

Figure 5-22A. This is an example of T-wave oversensing during exercise. Note that the actual heart rate is just above 100 bpm while the ICD sensed a rate of 223 bpm. The EGM also shows a relatively large T wave. Analysis of R-R interval in therapy history showed an abrupt onset of short R-R, mimicking a true onset of a VT (Figure 5-22B).

Episode 4	R-R Intervals								
	Date 03-JAN-00			Time 03:48			Type Spontaneous		
Onset	568 --	566 --	559 --	555 --	549 --	549 --	541 --	410 --	150 VF	523 VS
	537 VS	535 VS	535 VS	533 VS	535 VS	535 VS	320 VF	230 VF	242 VF	293 VF
	225 VF	307 VF	223 VF	309 VF						
Initial Detection	355 VS	199 VF	301 VF	223 VF						
Attempt 1 VF Shk 1	525 VS Chrg	539 VS Chrg	260 VF Chrg	291 VF Chrg	256 VF Chrg	283 VF Chrg	523 VS Chrg	537 VS Chrg	324 VF Chrg	211 VF Chrg
	535 VS Chrg	541 VS Chrg	535 VS Chrg	535 VS Chrg	18 --					
Redetection	521 VS	541 VS	537 VS	543 VS	545 VS	549 VS	549 VS	551 VS	447 VS	137 VF
	523 VS	561 VS	563 VS	568 VS	572 VS	566 VS	570 VS	574 VS	572 VS	
	End of Episode									

* All energies reported as stored.
End of Report

Figure 5-22B. R-R interval history of the event in Figure 5-22A. Note the abrupt onset of short coupling interval of 320 ms, mimicking VT.

QRS double sensing is another cause of inappropriate shock although it is relatively uncommon. It can occur in the case of a wide-QRS complex. Immediately after the blanking period (nominally set, non-programmable, at 120-140 ms), normal sensing resumes. Thus, in the presence of a wide-QRS, there is a possibility of double sensing. Fortunately, it is a quite rare occurrence, as the initial sensing would normally occur within (and not at the onset of) the QRS complex where the slew rate is highest, and hence, only an extremely wide QRS complex would pose the risk for double sensing. Although, again, such phenomenon should have been noted during implantation, deterioration in cardiac status and chronic antiarrhythmic drug use can alter the QRS significantly, producing delayed QRS-complex widening. Furthermore, the use-dependence effect of antiarrhythmic drug may cause significant QRS-widening during sinus tachycardia, which would have been noted only if the patient is exercised. Thus, to asses the possibility of QRS-complex double sensing, one should perform a resting and/or exercise electrocardiogram along with marker channel or beep-o-gram analysis.

Pacemaker stimulus can cause oversensing especially if the pacemaker is not an integral part of the ICD; and of a particular concern is a unipolar pacemaker or a pacemaker that may revert to unipolar after a shock (a non-dedicated bipolar pacemaker). Analysis of the marker channel or beep-o-gram during a paced event can identify this problem. To assess the worst case scenario, the patient should be paced 100% (in the VOO or DOO mode) at the highest output. Because such negative device interaction is also analyzed at implantation, it would be unusual to see it in late follow up. If present, one should look for lead dislodgment or migration.

Oversensing of other external stimuli should also be considered in troubleshooting inappropriate therapy. The patient might have been inadvertently exposed to a strong external electromagnetic force. Nowadays, where most ICDs are adequately shielded to external stimuli, such occurrences are rare. However, if an inappropriate shock from an external source is suspected, one must obtain a detail history of the events and circumstances leading to the shock and carefully analyze the event EGM and marker channel for the presence of high frequency signals.

As in the case of pacemakers, oversensing with ICDs can be caused inappropriate lead function, such as dislodgment or insulation damage. The sensing lead should be interrogated for changes or marked drop in its pacing impedance and its overall integrity should be examined radiographically. If an intermittent problem is suspected, the lead should be "stressed" by having the patient perform body movements, including reproducing the postures leading to the inappropriate shocks while recording the lead's EGM and marker channel or performing the beep-o-gram.

A rather common occurrence of oversensing problem is diaphragmatic sensing. This appears to be particularly common with the CPI/Guidant Endotak leads. Such oversensing produces fine high-frequency noise that can usually be detected and reproduced with diaphragmatic maneuvers while continuously recording the EGM (Figure 5-23).

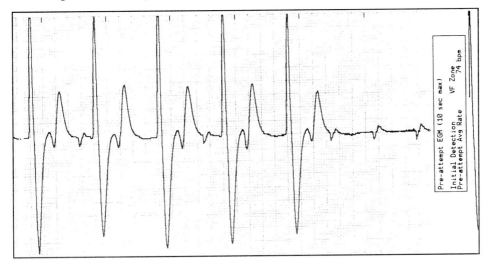

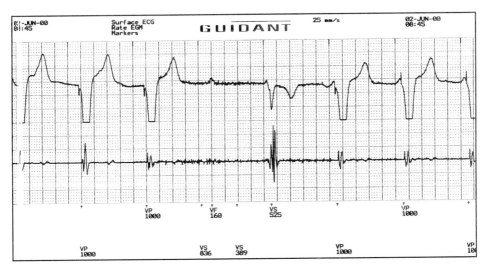

Figure 5-23. An example of diaphragmatic oversensing. The top panel shows the pre-shock EGM whereby baseline noise was noted and ventricular pacing ceased, indicating an oversensing problem. The lower panel shows reproduction of noise and multiple V-sensing (VS-VF-VS) by deep inspiration, consistent with diaphragmatic oversensing.

Therapy Failure

Another problem, which is potentially more serious is therapy failure. In the event of syncope or cardiac arrest, the history is frequently incomplete because the patient had lost consciousness and developed a lapse in his/her memory; hence, it would be difficult to ascertain whether or not therapy had been delivered. In such a case, the patient or family member would commonly assume that the device had failed to deliver the appropriate therapy. The physician should first differentiate whether there was indeed failure to deliver a therapy or whether it was a case of ineffective therapy. This would have been difficult if not impossible to confirm with the earlier generation ICDs that are not equipped with a stored EGM feature and one would have had to rely on the shock count tally. With the newer ICDs, the stored event data or therapy history would elucidate whether the device failed to recognize the arrhythmia or failed to terminate it after exhausting all programmed therapy.

Failure to Deliver Therapy

Failure to deliver therapy can be caused by sensing failure, inadequate programming or inadvertent device deactivation. Interrogation of the device would immediately clarify whether the device was active and whether the detection parameters were programmed adequately. Once these have been ruled out, the sensing function of the device should be examined.

In spite of the many safety features that are built in to avoid inadvertent device deactivation, there have been cases of sudden death of ICD patients with their units turned off.[129] With the CPI unit, permanent deactivation can occur with exposure to a strong electromagnetic field for 30 seconds. This feature was a fixed (non-programmable) in their older unit. In the newer models, this feature is programmable; hence, if not activated, prolonged exposure to a magnet would not turn off the device. Many other devices can not be turned off permanently; however, their sensing mechanism can be "blinded" temporarily during exposure to a strong external electromagnetic stimulus.

Thus, in most cases, device deactivation is assumed to be due to erroneous programming. Other causes for device deactivation, albeit rare, are accelerated battery depletion and a shutdown mode, whereby self-deactivation occurs because the device detects the potential of unsafe or unreliable operation. Investigation of the possibility of such mechanical changes can be easily done through device interrogation. Troubleshooting of the likelihood of temporary or transient inadvertent device deactivation and its causes, on the other hand, is quite difficult, even after meticulous history taking.

A more common cause for failure to deliver therapy is inaccurate or inappropriate device programming. A common step in programming error is in the estimation of rate cut off. Difficulty with programming VT rate cut off is common in patients who are being treated with antiarrhythmic drugs, especially when the dose of the drug is being modified or combination drug therapy is implemented. In such cases, VT rate can constantly change and may escape detection intermittently (Figures 5-24A and 5-24B) or even totally.

The estimation of VT cycle length change with the use of antiarrhythmic drug is difficult if not impossible. The ideal method would be repeating VT induction after a significant change in antiarrhythmic drug therapy but even this method would not be conclusive either because it might not reveal all of the possible VT morphology that would occur clinically. The Biotronik detection scheme includes a "buffer" tachy-hysteresis zone that would allow inclusion of VT with CL harboring at the border zone and may be an ideal solution for such condition. This tachy-hysteresis zone is programmable between 10-200 ms

Fortunately, in most instances, a VT episode that is slower than the rate cut off is also usually too slow to cause immediate hemodynamic collapse. In the event of progressive hypotension, the VT would naturally accelerate and eventually satisfy the detection rate cut off. Nevertheless, a prolonged episode of tachycardia can cause significant clinical consequences, especially in a patient with coronary artery disease.

ID#	Date/Time	V. Cycle	Duration	Reason
36	Jan 27 13:57:24	440 ms	7 beats	Non-Sustained
35	Jan 27 13:57:11	440 ms	14 beats	Non-Sustained
34	Jan 27 13:57:06	440 ms	10 beats	Non-Sustained
33	Jan 27 13:57:02	440 ms	10 beats	Non-Sustained
32	Jan 27 13:56:57	440 ms	10 beats	Non-Sustained
31	Jan 27 13:56:49	440 ms	6 beats	Non-Sustained
30	Jan 27 13:56:01	440 ms	6 beats	Non-Sustained
29	Jan 27 13:55:55	430 ms	10 beats	Non-Sustained
28	Jan 27 13:55:50	430 ms	10 beats	Non-Sustained
27	Jan 27 13:55:44	430 ms	10 beats	Non-Sustained
26	Jan 27 13:55:40	440 ms	10 beats	Non-Sustained
25	Jan 27 13:55:29	440 ms	10 beats	Non-Sustained
24	Jan 27 13:55:26	440 ms	7 beats	Non-Sustained
23	Jan 27 13:54:41	430 ms	6 beats	Non-Sustained
22	Jan 27 13:53:40	430 ms	6 beats	Non-Sustained
21	Jan 27 12:01:53	430 ms	7 beats	Non-Sustained
20	Jan 17 10:10:30	370 ms	6 beats	Non-Sustained
9	Jan 12 11:46:17	350 ms	6 beats	Non-Sustained

Figure 5-24A. Therapy history data from a patient who experienced a 2-hour episode of tachycardia without receiving therapy. VT detection rate was at 450 ms. Episodes 21 - 36 contained "NSVT" at CL of 430 and 440 ms. This is a typical scenario of a slow VT that harbors right near the detection rate cut off. This is further illustrated in Figure 5-24B.

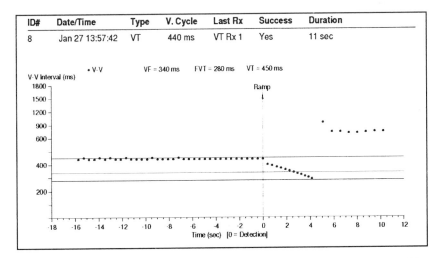

ID#	Date/Time	Type	V. Cycle	Last Rx	Success	Duration
8	Jan 27 13:57:42	VT	440 ms	VT Rx 1	Yes	11 sec

Figure 5-24B. The same VT episode as in Figure 5-24A that eventually stayed under 450 ms CL and was appropriately detected and successfully treated with a single ramp ATP. Note how closely the VT CL stayed under the detection cut off rate.

Another scenario that can cause failure in therapy delivery is the erroneous programming of the device to a "monitor-only" mode, which is now considerably uncommon as the newer units are equipped with safety and warning features to prevent such a mishap. In some older models, such as the CPI Ventak PRX I and II units, the programming step for the therapy scheme is separate from the one for "Device Status" that includes the choices of "MONITOR+THERAPY", "MONITOR", or "OFF". Thus, selection and programming of therapy scheme selection would not automatically program the device to implement the therapy without programming the status of the device. In most current ICD models, a "monitor-only" option is not available in the high-rate zone (VF zone). Furthermore, in most models now, the choices of therapy scheme would not be available without first programming the therapy to be "ON". Simple interrogation of the device can readily identify and correct these problems.

Current devices are equipped with many advanced features to enhance discrimination between VT and supraventricular arrhythmias. However, the discriminatory method is frequently based only on the relationship between the ventricular and atrial electrogram. Thus, some VT could be misinterpreted as a supraventricular tachycardia and would not receive the appropriate therapy. Furthermore, some patients may present with a wide spectrum of VT requiring a complex tiered-therapy programming with various anti-tachycardia pacing schemes. Such a situation may prolong delivery of a shock. Complex discriminatory and tiered-therapy schemes may delay shock therapy. In these cases, it would be advisable to program a safety feature by which the patient would receive a definitive, shock without going through a prolonged episode. The presence of this safety therapy feature should be checked if a "therapy failure" is suspected.

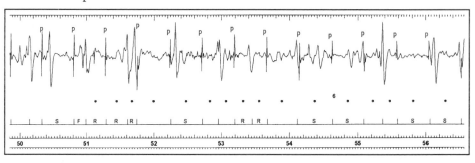

Figure 5-18. This tracing shows a recording during "fine" VF which was not sensed by a separate pacemaker unit. Thus, pacing (marked by "P"s) at maximum rate of 120 bpm (which was driven by motion from CPR) occurred, which in turn reset the automatic gain setting and caused undersensing of the tachyarrhythmia. Of note, the pacemaker was a dedicated bipolar unit but, in contrast to the episode shown in Figure 5-15B, the pacing output could be noted clearly.

Under-sensing tachyarrhythmia can lead to failure in therapy delivery. One common scenario is an under-sensing of fine ventricular fibrillation (VF). If this is suspected, a repeat measurement of the intrinsic R-wave and analysis of the under-sensed rhythm should be performed. The possibility of a negative interaction with a separate pacemaker unit should also be entertained. Thus, in the event of the pacemaker's failure to recognize VF, brady pacing might occur and the resultant pacing stimulus artifact might, in turn, "fool" and reset the sensing of the ICD unit (Figure 5-25).

If the arrhythmia was anything other than VF, one should investigate the function of the sensing mechanism, including the settings and lead integrity. The stored EGM and marker channels would not be helpful in suspected under-sensing, simply because this function would not have been triggered in the absence of sensing; hence the elucidation of under-sensing would frequently require induction of VT in the electrophysiology laboratory. Analysis of lead integrity should include the evaluation of R-wave stability, measurement of lead impedance, and investigation for structural discontinuity on radiographic study.

Ineffective Therapy

The other cause for therapy failure is the delivery of ineffective therapy, in which case, the device has terminated further attempts at treating the arrhythmia because it has exhausted all programmed therapies for that event. The stored EGM and therapy history would be most helpful in troubleshooting this scenario.

In the case of an ineffective shock, one should pay particular attention to the delivered energy. In the event of lead damage, the patient might have not received the full stored energy if the lead impedance is very low (due to insulation break) or extremely high (due to lead fracture). This should then be confirmed with examination of the lead radiographically and lead integrity testing, using a low-energy or full-energy shock.

The other possibility is an arrhythmia that is refractory to the therapy. It should be noted that defibrillation success is only a statistical function and some VF may be refractory to even full, high-energy shock.[76,130] Thus, patients with a high "defibrillation threshold" should be carefully re-evaluated for the possibility of failure due to inadequate defibrillation.[76] However, it would also be statistically possible that a VF is refractory to the full ICD shock energy even in patients who do not have a high DFT. Another situation is a rising DFT due to disease progression, decompensated congestive heart failure, active ischemia, or antiarrhythmic drug effect. The clinical history, especially changes in antiarrhythmic drug regimen should be carefully reviewed. Yet another cause for a refractory VF is a delay in therapy. If the VF is a result of a VT that degenerated after multiple attempts of antitachycardia pacing therapy, the patient might have been in a prolonged compromised hemodynamic state when therapy for VF was delivered. The appropriateness of the programmed ATP may need to be re-evaluated in the electrophysiology laboratory.

Finally, there is the possibility that therapy was effective for terminating arrhythmia but the patient subsequently died from other cardiac factors. In the evaluation of ICD patients reported to have sudden death, it was noted that in some patients with protracted arrhythmia and congestive heart failure, the ICD was finally successful at terminating VT/VF but the victims never recovered.

ICD Proarrhythmia

Although rare, ICD proarrhythmia has been noted to occur. The combination of inappropriate therapy and the induction of a more malignant arrhythmia can result into serious circumstances. There have been a few reports of death from such an "ICD proarrhythmia". In our experience, we have noted at least one documented event where the patient received a shock therapy for an SVT, which then induced VT which further degenerated into VF with the subsequent shocks, which persisted after all therapies have been exhausted.

There are several key factors involved in the proclivity of such a scenario. First of all, it is initiated by inappropriate detection, which would be more likely to occur in the absence detection enhancements. With present ICDs, this "trigger" has hopefully been diminished. The second factor is the induction of VT or VF by the inappropriate therapy. Unfortunately, such an incident is not uncommon. Overdrive pacing (ATP) can certainly induce VT, and a shock that falls within the vulnerable period can induce VF. Such induction is probably more common with a shock of a low or intermediate strength that would fall within the lower and upper limit of vulnerability. The final and most serious factor is the failure of the device to terminate the induced VT or VF. Such a failure is probably more likely to occur with older ICD models, where, typically, only up to four successive therapies are available for any arrhythmia episode; and thus, there would be two or three remaining therapies after the induction of VT or VF. In the newer models, more therapies are available and furthermore, with the use of biphasic waveform, a maximum-energy shock would have greater margin of efficacy compared to the monophasic shocks utilized in the older ICDs.

In summary, troubleshooting ICD requires a thorough history taking and device interrogation. Although, unquestionably, the event and therapy history is the most useful and important information, other device functions should be carefully analyzed, including the sense-pace and high-voltage lead properties, detection and therapy parameters, and possible interaction with other implanted device or external environment. Sometimes, radiographic examination may be helpful at identifying lead(s) integrity. Finally, arrhythmia induction and other maneuvers may be necessary to induce or unmask problems that may occur only intermittently.

> **Trouble shooting ICD requires thorough examination of the device, including assessment of electrophysiologic parameters and review of therapy history**

Table 5-3. Troubleshooting

Suspected Problem	Troubleshooting Steps

Suspected Inappropriate Shocks

Asymptomatic tachyarrhythmia	Analysis of event EGM (R-R interval and morphology)
Asymptomatic VT	Analysis of VT rate and duration, comparison of the event with patient's previous VT, and a review of the patient's previous history with respect to tolerance to VT
Other tachyarrhythmias	Analysis of event EGM and (if available) its atrial channel; and the outcome of the shock
Sinus tachycardia	Analysis of event EGM, particularly with respect to onset and morphology and attempt at reproducing the event with an exercise stress test.
T-wave and P-wave oversensing	Analysis of marker channel or beep-o-gram at various heart rates; re-evaluation of R-wave signal strength and stability, re-evaluation of lead position.
QRS doublesensing	Analysis of ECG along with intracardiac EGM and marker channel; reviewing patient's history with respect to antiarrhythmic drug regimen
Pacemaker-stimulus oversensing	Analysis of marker channel or beep-o-gram during a 100% paced event (DOO or VOO mode) at maximum pacemaker output.
Oversensing of external stimuli	Analysis of event EGM for high frequency signal and review of history of circumstances leading to the shock
Lead malfunction	Analysis of lead function in terms of pacing, sensing and impedance parameters and lead integrity

Suspected Therapy Failure

Inadvertent device deactivation	Device interrogation and history
Inaccurate device programming	Device interrogation
Prolonged delay in therapy	Analyze complexity of programmed features, such as complex discriminatory steps and detection enhancements, detection duration and inadvertent omission of a safety back up therapy
Sensing interference	Analysis of R-wave sensing and possible negative interactions with pacemaker.
Inadequate shock output	Interrogation of delivered therapy and analysis of high-voltage lead integrity including impedance.
Refractory arrhythmia	Evaluation of defibrillation threshold (DFT) and review of history, including progression of heart disease and changes in antiarrhythmic drug regimen.

References

1. Hauser R, Almquist A, and Kallinen L. Occult failure of implantable cardioverter defibrillator systems. PACE, 1999;**22**(6(II)):A-141.

2. Poole JE, Bardy GH, Dolack GL, *et al.* Serial defibrillation threshold measures in man: a prospective controlled study. J Cardiovasc Electrophysiol, 1995;**6**(1):19-25.

3. Guarnieri T, Levine JH, Veltri EP, *et al.* Success of chronic defibrillation and the role of antiarrhythmic drugs with the automatic implantable cardioverter/defibrillator. Am J Cardiol, 1987;**60**(13):1061-1064.

4. Huang SK, Tan de Guzman WL, Chenarides JG, *et al.* Effects of long-term amiodarone therapy on the defibrillation threshold and the rate of shocks of the implantable cardioverter-defibrillator. Am Heart J, 1991;**122**(3 Pt 1):720-727.

5. Jung W, Manz M, and Luderitz B. Effects of antiarrhythmic drugs on defibrillation threshold in patients with the implantable cardioverter defibrillator. Pacing Clin Electrophysiol, 1992;**15**(4 Pt 3):645-648.

6. Manz M, Jung W, and Luderitz B. Interactions between drugs and devices: experimental and clinical studies. Am Heart J, 1994;**127**(4 Pt 2):978-984.

7. Pycha C, Calabrese JR, Gulledge AD, *et al.* Patient and spouse acceptance and adaptation to implantable cardioverter defibrillators. Cleve Clin J Med, 1990;**57**(5):441-444.

8. Sneed NV, Finch NJ, and Michel Y. The effect of psychosocial nursing intervention on the mood state of patients with implantable cardioverter defibrillators and their caregivers. Prog Cardiovasc Nurs, 1997;**12**(2):4-14.

9. Jung W and Luderitz B. Quality of life and driving in recipients of the implantable cardioverter-defibrillator. Am J Cardiol, 1996;**78**(5A):51-56.

10. Hegel MT, Griegel LE, Black C, *et al.* Anxiety and depression in patients receiving implanted cardioverter- defibrillators: a longitudinal investigation. Int J Psychiatry Med, 1997;**27**(1):57-69.

11. Craney JM, Mandle CL, Munro BH, *et al.* Implantable cardioverter defibrillators: physical and psychosocial outcomes. Am J Crit Care, 1997;**6**(6):445-451.

12. Dunbar SB, Kimble LP, Jenkins LS, *et al.* Association of mood disturbance and arrhythmia events in patients after cardioverter defibrillator implantation. Depress Anxiety, 1999;**9**(4):163-168.

13. Schuster PM, Phillips S, Dillon DL, *et al.* The psychosocial and physiological experiences of patients with an implantable cardioverter defibrillator. Rehabil Nurs, 1998;**23**(1):30-37.

14. Sears SF, Jr., Todaro JF, Lewis TS, *et al.* Examining the psychosocial impact of implantable cardioverter defibrillators: a literature review. Clin Cardiol, 1999;**22**(7):481-489.

15. Weiss R, Ostrow E, Malkin R, *et al.* Low defibrillationenergy dose (LoDED) trial:is a five-joule defibrillation safety margin enough? Circulation, 1999;**100**(18):I-786.

16. Fries R, Jung J, Schieffer H, *et al.* Relation between the number of failed antitachycardia pacing attempts and the back-up shock efficacy in patients with implantable cardioverter-defibrillator. PACE, 1998;**21**(4(II)):952.

17. Pfitzner P, Trappe HJ, Fieguth HG, *et al.* [Experiences with the new cardioverter-defibrillator Ventak PRxII]. Z Kardiol, 1995;**84**(4):275-283.

18. Fiek M, Hoffmann E, Dorwarth U, *et al.* [Long-term efficacy of antitachycardia pacing for treatment of ventricular tachycardia in patients with implantable cardioverter/defibrillator]. Z Kardiol, 1999;**88**(10):815-822.

19. Nasir N, Jr., Pacifico A, Doyle TK, *et al.* Spontaneous ventricular tachycardia treated by antitachycardia pacing. Cadence Investigators. Am J Cardiol, 1997;**79**(6):820-822.

20. Schaumann A, Poppinga A, Gonska B, *et al.* Efficacy of antitachycardia pacing in 160 patients with a history of ventricular fibrillation. Circulation, 1999;**100**(18):I-571.

21. Josephson ME, Horowitz LN, Farshidi A, *et al.* Recurrent sustained ventricular tachycardia. 1. Mechanisms. Circulation, 1978;**57**(3):431-440.

22. Schaumann A, Poppinga A, vonzurMuehlen F, *et al.* Antitachycardia pacing for ventricular tachycardias above and below 200 bpm: a prospective study for ramp vs scan mode. PACE, 1997;**20**(4(II)):1108.

23. Fiek M, Dorwarth U, Muller D, *et al.* Predictors of efficacy of antitachycardia pacing for treatment of ventricular tachycardia in patients with implantable cardioverter/defibrillator (ICD). PACE, 1999;**22**(6(II)):A-144.

24. Marrouche N, Gerritse B, and Brachmann J. The efficacy of the anti-tachycardia pacing therapy in implantable cardioverter defibrillator patients depending on the average cycle length of the ventricular tachycardia. PACE, 1999;**22**(6(II)):A-140.

25. Fries R, Heisel A, Jung J, *et al.* Antitachycardia pacing in patients with implantable cardioverter-defibrillator: inverse circadian variation of therapy success and acceleration. PACE, 1997;**20**(4(II)):1107.

26. Liem LB, Mason DM, Jr., and Swerdlow CD. Strength-interval relation for ventricular functional refractoriness. Am J Cardiol, 1988;**61**(1):88-92.

27. Fiek M, Dorwarth U, Muller D, *et al.* Which antitachycardia pacing mode is superior fo the treatment of ventricular tachycardia in patients with implantable cardioverter defibrillator (ICD)? PACE, 1999;**22**(6(II)):A-140.

28. Josephson ME, Horowitz LN, Farshidi A, *et al.* Sustained ventricular tachycardia: evidence for protected localized reentry. Am J Cardiol, 1978;**42**(3):416-424.

29. Josephson ME, Horowitz LN, Farshidi A, *et al.* Recurrent sustained ventricular tachycardia. 4. Pleomorphism. Circulation, 1979;**59**(3):459-468.

30. Thamasett S, Grossmann G, Kochs M, *et al.* Only seven antitachycardia pacing attempts with an implantable cardioverter defibrillator are necessary to terminate a ventricular tachycardia. PACE, 1999;**22**(6(II)):A-139.

31. Ciccone JM, Saksena S, Shah Y, *et al.* A prospective randomized study of the clinical efficacy and safety of transvenous cardioversion for termination of ventricular tachycardia. Circulation, 1985;**71**(3):571-578.

32. Vergara G, Disertori M, Inama G, *et al.* [Sustained ventricular tachycardia: low-energy transcatheter internal cardioversion. Efficacy, reliability and tolerance in comparison with ventricular burst]. G Ital Cardiol, 1985;**15**(9):862-872.

33. Bardy GH, Poole JE, Kudenchuk PJ, *et al.* A prospective randomized repeat-crossover comparison of antitachycardia pacing with low-energy cardioversion. Circulation, 1993;**87**(6):1889-1896.

34. Saksena S, Chandran P, Shah Y, *et al.* Comparative efficacy of transvenous cardioversion and pacing in patients with sustained ventricular tachycardia: a prospective, randomized, crossover study. Circulation, 1985;**72**(1):153-160.

35. Winkle RA, Stinson EB, Bach SM, Jr., *et al.* Measurement of cardioversion/defibrillation thresholds in man by a truncated exponential waveform and an apical patch-superior vena caval spring electrode configuration. Circulation, 1984;**69**(4):766-771.

36. Lauer MR, Young C, Liem LB, *et al.* Ventricular fibrillation induced by low-energy shocks from programmable implantable cardioverter-defibrillators in patients with coronary artery disease. Am J Cardiol, 1994;**73**(8):559-563.

37. Neuzner J, *Programmierung zusatzlicher erkenennungskriterien*, in *Implantierbare Kardioverter-Defibrillatoren*, D. Wietholt, L. Ulbricht, and H. Gulker, Editors. 1997, Georg Thieme Verlag: Stuttgart. p. 175-185.

38. Brugada J, Mont L, Figueiredo M, *et al.* Enhanced detection criteria in implantable defibrillators. J Cardiovasc Electrophysiol, 1998;**9**(3):261-268.

39. Schaumann A, Poppinga A, Gonska B, *et al.* Long term efficacy of algorithms for discrimination of ventricular from supraventricular tachycardias in a single lead cardioverter-defibrillator. Circulation, 1999;**100**(18):I-569.

40. Swerdlow CD, Chen PS, Kass RM, *et al.* Discrimination of ventricular tachycardia from sinus tachycardia and atrial fibrillation in a tiered-therapy cardioverter-defibrillator. J Am Coll Cardiol, 1994;**23**(6):1342-1355.

41. Nanthakumar K, Newman D, Gunderson B, *et al.* A sudden onset algorithm differentiates sinus tachycardia from ventricular tachycardia in implantable defibrillators. Circulation, 1999;**100**(18):I-570.

42. Nanthakumar K, Deno K, Paquette M, *et al.* Is there an ideal stability algorithm to distinguish ventricular tachycardia from atrial fibrillation. Circulation, 1999;**100**(18):I-570.

43. Ruetz L, Bardy G, Mitchell L, *et al.* Clinical evaluation of electrogramwidth measurements for automatic detection of ventricular tachycardia. PACE, 1996;**19**(4(II)):582.

44. Barold HS, Newby KH, Tomassoni G, *et al.* Prospective evaluation of new and old criteria to discriminate between supraventricular and ventricular tachycardia in implantable defibrillators. Pacing Clin Electrophysiol, 1998;**21**(7):1347-1355.

45. Swerdlow C, Mandel W, and Ziccardi T. Effects of rate and procainamide on electrogram width measured by a tier-therapy implantable cardioverter-defibrillator. PACE, 1996;**19**(4(II)):734.

46. Duru F, Schonbeck M, Luscher TF, *et al.* The potential for inappropriate ventricular tachycardia confirmation using the Intracardiac Electrogram (EGM) Width Criterion. Pacing Clin Electrophysiol, 1999;**22**(7):1039-1046.

47. Herwig S, Jung W, Wolpert C, *et al.* First result with a new morphology criterion dor discrimination of supraventricular and ventricular tachycardias. J Am Coll Cardiol, 2000:127A.

48. Schulte B, Sperzel J, Schwarz T, *et al.* Temporal and exercise-related stability of a new "morphology-based" arrhythmia detection parameter in implantable defibrillators. PACE, 1999;**22**(4(II)):823.

49. Wilkoff B, Gillberg J, Hillman S, *et al.* Clinical experiencewith detection of spontaneous ventricular arrhythmias by a new dual chamber defibrillator in a multicenter study. Circulation, 1998;**98**(17):I-289.

50. Wilkoff B, Kuhlkamp V, Gillberg J, *et al.* Performance of a dual chamber detection akgorithm (PR Logic) based onthe worldwide Gem DR clinical results. PACE, 1999;**22**(4(II)):720.

51. Hug B, Hambrecht R, Hindricks G, *et al.* Safety and performance of a newdualchamber implantable cardioverter-defibrillator (ICD): resultsfrom a European multicenter study. J Am Coll Cardiol, 1999:115A.

52. Kuhlkamp V, Dornberger V, Suchalla R, *et al.* Specificity and sensitivity of a detection algorithm using patterns, AV-association and rate analysis for the differentiation of supraventricular tachyarrhythmias and ventricular tachyarrhythmias. PACE, 1999;**22**(4(II)):823.

53. Sadoul N, Chauvin M, Leenhardt A, *et al.* Usefulness of dual chamber detection algorithm in ICD. Initial clinical experience. Circulation, 1996;**94**(8):I-321.

54. Jung W, Wolpert C, Spehl S, *et al.* Classification algorithm for discrimination of ventricular tachycardia from supraventricular tachycardia. PACE, 1998;**21**(4(II)):402.

55. Jung W, Wolpert C, Spehl S, *et al.* Prospective evaluation of a new arrhythmiaclassification algorithm for discrimination of ventricular tachycardia from supraventricular tachycardia. PACE, 1999;**22**(4(II)):890.

56. Revishvili A. Dual-chamber implantable cardioverter-defibrillator with active discriminationof supraventricular tachycardia. Progress in Biomedical Research, 1999;**2**:166-171.

57. Pinski S, Haw J, and Trohman R. Usefulness of a dynamic post-pace ventricular blanking period in dual-chamber, rate-responsiveimplantable defibrillators. PACE, 1999;**22**(4(II)):897.

58. Karolyi L, Armbruster T, Hilbel T, *et al.* Analysis of critical Rr sequences prior to spontaneous ventricular arrhythmia in patients with new implantable cardioverter-defibrillator. PACE, 1998;**21**(4(II)):968.

59. Perez-Castellano N, Arenal A, Gonzales S, *et al.* Mechanism of onset of spontaneous ventricular tachyarrhythmias. PACE, 1999;**22**(4(II)):838.

60. Dorwarth U, Koblbauer S, Fiek M, *et al.* Preventive pacing for ventricular tachyarrhythmias in patients with ICD: perspective for clinical application. PACE, 1999;**22**(4(II)):830.

61. Beatch GN, Dickenson DR, Wood RH, *et al.* Class III antiarrhythmic effects of LY-190147 on defibrillation threshold. J Cardiovasc Pharmacol, 1996;**27**(2):218-225.

62. Dorian P, Newman D, Sheahan R, *et al.* d-Sotalol decreases defibrillation energy requirements in humans: a novel indication for drug therapy. J Cardiovasc Electrophysiol, 1996;**7**(10):952-961.

63. Qi XQ, Newman D, and Dorian P. Azimilide decreases defibrillation voltage requirements and increases spatial organization during ventricular fibrillation. J Interv Card Electrophysiol, 1999;**3**(1):61-67.

64. Singh BN. Sotalol: Current Status and Expanding Indications. J Cardiovasc Pharmacol Ther, 1999;**4**(1):49-65.

65. Spinelli W, Parsons RW, and Colatsky TJ. Effects of WAY-123,398, a new class III antiarrhythmic agent, on cardiac refractoriness and ventricular fibrillation threshold in anesthetized dogs: a comparison with UK-68798, E-4031, and dl-sotalol. J Cardiovasc Pharmacol, 1992;**20**(6):913-922.

66. Wang M and Dorian P. DL and D sotalol decrease defibrillation energy requirements. Pacing Clin Electrophysiol, 1989;**12**(9):1522-1529.

67. Davis DR, Beatch GN, Dickenson DR, *et al.* Dofetilide enhances shock-induced extension of refractoriness and lowers defibrillation threshold. Can J Cardiol, 1999;**15**(2):193-200.

68. Wesley RC, Jr., Farkhani F, Morgan D, *et al.* Ibutilide: enhanced defibrillation via plateau sodium current activation. Am J Physiol, 1993;**264**(4 Pt 2):H1269-1274.

69. Dorian P and Newman D. Tedisamil increases coherence during ventricular fibrillation and decreases defibrillation energy requirements. Cardiovasc Res, 1997;**33**(2):485-494.

70. Ujhelyi MR, Schur M, Frede T, *et al.* Differential effects of lidocaine on defibrillation threshold with monophasic versus biphasic shock waveforms. Circulation, 1995;**92**(6):1644-1650.

71. Deeb GM, Hardesty RL, Griffith BP, *et al.* The effects of cardiovascular drugs on the defibrillation threshold and the pathological effects on the heart using an automatic implantable defibrillator. Ann Thorac Surg, 1983;**35**(4):361-366.

72. Babbs CF, Yim GK, Whistler SJ, *et al.* Elevation of ventricular defibrillation threshold in dogs by antiarrhythmic drugs. Am Heart J, 1979;**98**(3):345-350.

73. Murakawa Y, Sezaki K, Inoue H, *et al.* Shock-induced refractory period extension and pharmacologic modulation of defibrillation threshold. J Cardiovasc Pharmacol, 1994;**23**(5):822-825.

74.   Echt DS, Gremillion ST, Lee JT, *et al.* Effects of procainamide and lidocaine on defibrillation energy requirements in patients receiving implantable cardioverter defibrillator devices. J Cardiovasc Electrophysiol, 1994;**5**(9):752-760.

75.   Behrens S, Li C, and Franz MR. Effects of long-term amiodarone treatment on ventricular-fibrillation vulnerability and defibrillation efficacy in response to monophasic and biphasic shocks. J Cardiovasc Pharmacol, 1997;**30**(4):412-418.

76.   Epstein AE, Ellenbogen KA, Kirk KA, *et al.* Clinical characteristics and outcome of patients with high defibrillation thresholds. A multicenter study. Circulation, 1992;**86**(4):1206-1216.

77.   Jung W, Manz M, Pfeiffer D, *et al.* Effects of antiarrhythmic drugs on epicardial defibrillation energy requirements and the rate of defibrillator discharges. Pacing Clin Electrophysiol, 1993;**16**(1 Pt 2):198-201.

78.   Kuhlkamp V, Mewis C, Suchalla R, *et al.* Effect of amiodarone and sotalol on the defibrillation threshold in comparison to patients without antiarrhythmic drug treatment. Int J Cardiol, 1999;**69**(3):271-279.

79.   Natale A, Jones DL, Kleinstiver PW, *et al.* Effects of flecainide on defibrillation threshold in pigs. J Cardiovasc Pharmacol, 1993;**21**(4):573-577.

80.   Hernandez R, Mann DE, Breckinridge S, *et al.* Effects of flecainide on defibrillation thresholds in the anesthetized dog. J Am Coll Cardiol, 1989;**14**(3):777-781.

81.   Montenero AS, Bombardieri G, Barilaro C, *et al.* Intravenous propafenone reduces energy requirements for defibrillation in pigs. Cardiologia, 1990;**35**(4):291-294.

82.   Echt DS, Black JN, Barbey JT, *et al.* Evaluation of antiarrhythmic drugs on defibrillation energy requirements in dogs. Sodium channel block and action potential prolongation. Circulation, 1989;**79**(5):1106-1117.

83.   Kerber RE, Pandian NG, Jensen SR, *et al.* Effect of lidocaine and bretylium on energy requirements for transthoracic defibrillation: experimental studies. J Am Coll Cardiol, 1986;**7**(2):397-405.

84.   Sato S, Tsuji MH, and Naito H. Mexiletine has no effect on defibrillation energy requirements in dogs. Pacing Clin Electrophysiol, 1994;**17**(12 Pt 1):2279-2284.

85.   Sato S and Imagawa N. Effects of lidocaine and mexiletine on defibrillation energy requirements in animals treated with flecainide. Resuscitation, 1998;**36**(3):175-180.

86.   Chauvin M, Crenner F, and Brechenmacher C. Interaction between permanent cardiac pacing and electrocautery: the significance of electrode position. Pacing Clin Electrophysiol, 1992;**15**(11 Pt 2):2028-2033.

87.   Levine PA, Balady GJ, Lazar HL, *et al.* Electrocautery and pacemakers: management of the paced patient subject to electrocautery. Ann Thorac Surg, 1986;**41**(3):313-317.

88.   Chin MC, Rosenqvist M, Lee MA, *et al.* The effect of radiofrequency catheter ablation on permanent pacemakers: an experimental study. Pacing Clin Electrophysiol, 1990;**13**(1):23-29.

89.   Holmes DR, Jr., Hayes DL, Gray JE, *et al.* The effects of magnetic resonance imaging on implantable pulse generators. Pacing Clin Electrophysiol, 1986;**9**(3):360-370.

90.   Chung MK, Streem SB, Ching E, *et al.* Effects of extracorporeal shock wave lithotripsy on tiered therapy implantable cardioverter defibrillators. Pacing Clin Electrophysiol, 1999;**22**(5):738-742.

91.   Rasmussen MJ, Hayes DL, Vlietstra RE, *et al.* Can transcutaneous electrical nerve stimulation be safely used in patients with permanent cardiac pacemakers? Mayo Clin Proc, 1988;**63**(5):443-445.

92.   Rodriguez F, Filimonov A, Henning A, *et al.* Radiation-induced effects in multiprogrammable pacemakers and implantable defibrillators. Pacing Clin Electrophysiol, 1991;**14**(12):2143-2153.

93.   Carrillo R, Embrey M, Zebede J, *et al.* Should patints with pacemakers avoid the use of cellular telephones? A risk management research. PACE, 1997;**20**(4(II)):1150.

94.   Hayes D, Wang P, Estes N, *et al.* Effect of polarity configuration on pacemaker susceptibility to EMI from wireless phones. PACE, 1997;**20**(4(II)):1231.

95.   Gottlieb C, Sarter B, Coyne R, *et al.* Do transmmisions from cellular telephone antennas interfere with implantable cardioverter-defibrillator fucntion? PACE, 1997;**20**(4(II)):1167.

96.   Groh W, Boschee S, Engelstein E, *et al.* Interactionsbetween implanatable cardioverter defibrillators and electronic article surveillance systems. PACE, 1999;**22**(4(II)):724.

97.   Mathew P, Lewis C, Neglia J, *et al.* Interaction between electronic article surveillance systems and implantable defibrillators: insights from a fourth generation ICD [see comments]. Pacing Clin Electrophysiol, 1997;**20**(11):2857-2859.

98.   McIvor ME. Environmental electromagnetic interference from electronic article surveillance devices: interactions with an ICD. Pacing Clin Electrophysiol, 1995;**18**(12 Pt 1):2229-2230.

99.   McIvor ME, Reddinger J, Floden E, *et al.* Study of Pacemaker and Implantable Cardioverter Defibrillator Triggering by Electronic Article Surveillance Devices (SPICED TEAS) [see comments]. Pacing Clin Electrophysiol, 1998;**21**(10):1847-1861.

100. Tan K and Hinberg I. Can electronic article surveillancesystems affect implantable cardiac pacemakers and defibrillators? PACE, 1998;**21**(4(II)):960.

101. Fetter JG, Benditt DG, and Stanton MS. Electromagnetic interference from welding and motors on implantable cardioverter-defibrillators as tested in the electrically hostile work site. J Am Coll Cardiol, 1996;**28**(2):423-427.

102. Ahern T, Luckett C, Ehrlich S, et al. Use of bipolar electrocautery in patients with implantable cardioverter defibrillators: no reason to inactivate detection or therapies. PACE, 1999;**22**(4(II)):776.

103. Schumacher M, Olschewski M, and Schulgen G. Assessment of quality of life in clinical trials. Stat Med, 1991;**10**(12):1915-1930.

104. May CD, Smith PR, Murdock CJ, et al. The impact of the implantable cardioverter defibrillator on quality-of- life. Pacing Clin Electrophysiol, 1995;**18**(7):1411-1418.

105. Chevalier P, Verrier P, Kirkorian G, et al. Improved appraisal of the quality of life in patients with automatic implantable cardioverter defibrillator: a psychometric study. Psychother Psychosom, 1996;**65**(1):49-56.

106. Stankoweit B, Muthny FA, Block M, et al. [Quality of life after implantation of a cardioverter-defibrillator (ICD)--results of an empirical study of 132 ICD patients]. Z Kardiol, 1997;**86**(6):460-468.

107. Reid SS, McKinley S, and Nagy S. Outcomes, problems and quality of life with the implantable cardioverter defibrillator [In Process Citation]. Aust J Adv Nurs, 1999;**16**(4):14-19.

108. Vitale MB and Funk M. Quality of life in younger persons with an implantable cardioverter defibrillator. Dimens Crit Care Nurs, 1995;**14**(2):100-111.

109. Pycha C, Gulledge AD, Hutzler J, et al. Psychological responses to the implantable defibrillator: preliminary observations. Psychosomatics, 1986;**27**(12):841-845.

110. Vlay SC, Olson LC, Fricchione GL, et al. Anxiety and anger in patients with ventricular tachyarrhythmias. Responses after automatic internal cardioverter defibrillator implantation. Pacing Clin Electrophysiol, 1989;**12**(2):366-373.

111. Conti JB, Woodard DA, Tucker KJ, et al. Modification of patient driving behavior after implantation of a cardioverter defibrillator. Pacing Clin Electrophysiol, 1997;**20**(9 Pt 1):2200-2204.

112. Curtis AB, Conti JB, Tucker KJ, et al. Motor vehicle accidents in patients with an implantable cardioverter- defibrillator. J Am Coll Cardiol, 1995;**26**(1):180-184.

113. Craney JM and Powers MT. Factors related to driving in persons with an implantable cardioverter defibrillator. Prog Cardiovasc Nurs, 1995;**10**(3):12-17.

114. Anderson MH and Camm AJ. Legal and ethical aspects of driving and working in patients with an implantable cardioverter defibrillator. Am Heart J, 1994;**127**(4 Pt 2):1185-1193.

115. DiCarlo LA, Winston SA, Honoway S, et al. Driving restrictions advised by midwestern cardiologists implanting cardioverter defibrillators: present practices, criteria utilized, and compatibility with existing state laws. Pacing Clin Electrophysiol, 1992;**15**(8):1131-1136.

116. Finch NJ, Leman RB, Kratz JM, et al. Driving safety among patients with automatic implantable cardioverter defibrillators. Jama, 1993;**270**(13):1587-1588.

117. Larsen GC, Stupey MR, Walance CG, et al. Recurrent cardiac events in survivors of ventricular fibrillation or tachycardia. Implications for driving restrictions. Jama, 1994;**271**(17):1335-1339.

118. Bansch D, Brunn J, Castrucci M, et al. Syncope in patients with an implantable cardioverter-defibrillator: incidence, prediction and implications for driving restrictions. J Am Coll Cardiol, 1998;**31**(3):608-615.

119. Jung W, Anderson M, Camm AJ, et al. Recommendations for driving of patients with implantable cardioverter defibrillators. Study Group on 'ICD and Driving' of the Working Groups on Cardiac Pacing and Arrhythmias of the European Society of Cardiology. Eur Heart J, 1997;**18**(8):1210-1219.

120. Kowey PR, Marinchak RA, and Rials SJ. Things that go bang in the night [letter] [see comments]. N Engl J Med, 1992;**327**(26):1884.

121. Grimm W, Flores BF, and Marchlinski FE. Symptoms and electrocardiographically documented rhythm preceding spontaneous shocks in patients with implantable cardioverter- defibrillator. Am J Cardiol, 1993;**71**(16):1415-1418.

122. Maloney J, Masterson M, Khoury D, et al. Clinical performance of the implantable cardioverter defibrillator: electrocardiographic documentation of 101 spontaneous discharges. Pacing Clin Electrophysiol, 1991;**14**(2 Pt 2):280-285.

123. Dorian P, Newman D, Thibault B, et al. A randomized clinical trial of a standardized protocol for the prevention of inappropriate therapyusing a dual chamberimplantable cardioverter defibrillator. Circulation, 1999;**100**(18):I-786.

124. Lampert R, Rosenfeld L, McPherson C, et al. Initial single-center experience with an advanced third-generation investigational defibrillator. Pacing Clin Electrophysiol, 1996;**19**(12 Pt 1):2072-2082.

125.   Brugada J. Is inappropriate therapy a resolved issue with current implantable cardioverter defibrillators? Am J Cardiol, 1999;**83**(5B):40D-44D.

126.   Nayak HM, Tsao L, Santoni-Rugiu F, *et al.* A pitfall in using far-field bipolar electrograms in arrhythmia discrimination in a patient with an implantable cardioverter defibrillator. Pacing Clin Electrophysiol, 1997;**20**(11):2864-2866.

127.   Chapman PD and Troup P. The automatic implantable cardioverter-defibrillator: evaluating suspected inappropriate shocks. J Am Coll Cardiol, 1986;**7**(5):1075-1078.

128.   Ellenbogen KA, Wood MA, Stambler BS, *et al.* Measurement of ventricular electrogram amplitude during intraoperative induction of ventricular tachyarrhythmias. Am J Cardiol, 1992;**70**(11):1017-1022.

129.   Mosteller RD, Lehmann MH, Thomas AC, *et al.* Operative mortality with implantation of the automatic cardioverter- defibrillator. Am J Cardiol, 1991;**68**(13):1340-1345.

130.   Davy JM, Fain ES, Dorian P, *et al.* The relationship between successful defibrillation and delivered energy in open-chest dogs: reappraisal of the "defibrillation threshold" concept. Am Heart J, 1987;**113**(1):77-84.

CHAPTER 6

NEW FEATURES

The technology of ICD will undoubtedly continue to progress. The combination of constant demand for a better device and the rapidly growing technology would continue to fuel further improvement. Naturally, such progress will involve refinement of current features as well as implementation of newer ones. Improved understanding of arrhythmia mechanism and advancements in energy delivery will continue to lower the requirement for defibrillation; and coupled with progress in battery and capacitor technology, these will allow for further diminution of overall device size. Similarly, progress in lead technology will result in better sensing, pacing, and defibrillation; as well as allowing for special functions. Progress in leads technology will also likely to include the use of materials or composites that can better handle mechanical stress and biocompatible issues.

Even a greater progress will occur in the expansion of its therapeutic scope. In addition to providing therapy for brady- and tachyarrhythmias, the ICD would be likely to offer arrhythmia preventive unit and, eventually become a vehicle for other electrical-based therapeutic modalities. The current progress in multi-site pacing for ventricular resynchronization is just one example. In this chapter, some of these features will be discussed briefly.

Further Technological Refinement

The present ICD is a unit capable of delivering various therapies for tachyarrhythmia and bradyarrhythmia. With the addition of enhanced detection features and secondary bradycardia parameters, the unit has become a "complete" arrhythmia therapeutic device by current standards. As the size of the generator has become progressively smaller and will continue to do so in the near future, the device has also become increasingly more acceptable to the patients. The current ICD has therefore reached a new platform stage to which future units would be measured against.

While new features are being incorporated, pre-existing elements of the device will continue to be refined. These refinements, while not necessarily revolutionary, will continue to result in improved operation of the device. They include technological refinement of both the "hardware" and "software" components of the unit.

Improvement in Hardware Technology

Even though the ICD has become dramatically smaller in the past few years, there will be constant demand for further diminution of its overall size, shape and weight. Such a demand is fueled by a constant, albeit unrealistic comparison with pacemakers and the general expectation that all modern equipment will always get smaller. Nevertheless, ongoing technical research will undoubtedly result in the development of more "efficient" (for lack of a more practical technical term) batteries and capacitors, the components that occupy the greatest volume of the pulse generator. Combined with a better understanding of VT/VF mechanism and improved efficacy of defibrillation (and therefore a lower shock energy requirement), the technical advancements will result in the manufacturing of yet significantly smaller ICD.

Progress in Battery Technology

There has been little change in the material utilized in ICD batteries. The first material used as power source in the early models manufactured by Intec and a few generations afterwards was the lithium/vanadium oxide. This was then replaced by lithium/silver vanadium oxide (Li/SVO), which has been utilized since the late 1980s and shown to have reliable field performance (Chapter 3). Such a battery is faster in charging the capacitor than the conventional lithium iodide pacemaker battery but has less energy density.

The size of the battery depends largely on the configuration of its cells. Although there are many different models using different size and shape, they all share certain common design. The progress in this field includes more efficient packaging resulting in higher density cell and reshaping of the cell such that it would fit a rounded pulse generator.

The change from utilizing two batteries in series to a single large one has allowed for some but small reduction in pulse generator size. The one clinically notable effect of this change is the prolongation in charge time. However, improved efficiency in capacitor function has dramatically shortened the time to reach full charge in modern ICD units, even from a single battery. With the drawbacks of single battery being relatively minor, future units will likely stay with such a single battery operation.

Another ongoing consumer demand is improved longevity. This task is complicated by the fact that there is a progressive increase in device's features that use energy, such as telemetry and bradycardia pacing. These operations demand small but continuous amount of energy that the Li/SVO battery is not the most efficient for. The addition of a lithium oxide battery for bradycardia pacing component might be advantageous in terms of preserving the total device longevity but would add to its overall size. Thus, for a period of time, the overall advancement in ICD operation will involve these opposing factors that may result in the production of smaller unit but with variable longevity, depending on the complexity of its operation.

A more revolutionary development in the battery technology would likely involve the utilization of a different material for its power supply or a rechargeable unit. With similar ongoing progress in non-medical technology, such a change may not be too far in the future but its implementation may take longer in the medical field because of the rigorous constraints that typically involve in clinical experimentation.

Progress in Capacitor Technology

The capacitors also occupy a significant amount of space within the generator. Like the batteries, the capacitor occupies about one third of the ICD pulse generator.

The material used for ICD capacitor is the aluminum electrolytic because of its high energy density capacity. The typical ICD operating on a maximum delivery of 700 to 800 volts needs two of such capacitors because even with its high energy density, each of them can only have up to 500 volts operative capacity. The relative size and cylindrical shape of these capacitors as well as the extra sealing that is necessary to make them medically compatible also add to the bulkiness of ICD size. The use of alternative materials may reduce the size of the capacitor but progress in this field is met with difficulty in finding the appropriate substance.

Alteration in the capacitance, however, may improve defibrillation performance. It has been reported, for example, that capacitor using a 60-microfarad instead of the conventional 120-microfarad, defibrillates with lower stored energy.[1]

> There has been significant progress in battery and capacitor technology but improvements will continue to occur as a result of advancement in technology in general

Improvement in Lead Technology

Obviously, the ICD lead plays a major factor in the many features and performance of the ICD. In addition to delivering the defibrillation shock, the lead is the essential component in sensing and pacing and, in the future, other, more complex, functions. Thus, compared to pacemaker leads, the ICD lead contains more components and is therefore more bulky. Whether or not this is the reason for the relatively high incidence of lead failure in the early transvenous ICD system is not known. In one study, an 11.8% failure rate in 422 patients at 3.5-year follow up was noted.[2] In another study, the incidence of lead failure was lower, at 5.0% after 4 years, but became significantly higher, at 19.3% after 64 months[3], although this study combined the performance of epicardial and endocardial leads.

Progress in ICD leads has included numerous modifications. The change from thoracotomy to transvenous system has changed the design significantly. The major challenge of the transvenous lead was its limited surface area for its defibrillator electrode. The lower efficacy of defibrillation with the transvenous lead as compared to the efficacy of epicardial patch system was initially compensated with the use of additional defibrillation electrodes, such as the SVC and coronary sinus lead, and the subcutaneous patch and array. With the advent of biphasic waveform, however, a single transvenous lead alone is sufficient.

Another major disadvantage of the transvenous defibrillation is the non-uniform current density produced and the possibility of energy shunting by the blood, which has lower electrical impedance. Also a challenge in the use of transvenous lead is the incorporation of the sensing and pacing mechanism within the same defibrillation lead. This can cause some sensing problem after a high-energy shock because of the transient tissue dysfunction caused by the shock, especially at the tissue nearest the defibrillation electrode.

The advantage of the use of multiple lead or alternate lead position is now again investigated to assess if it can further lower the DFT. Various positions within the coronary sinus tributaries are being tested, showing indeed lowering of DFT as compared to the traditional right ventricular placement.[4-6] The left ventricular defibrillation alone offers reduction in DFT when compared to right ventricular alone, by 2 to 3 joules.[4] Biventricular defibrillation, however, offers further reduction of the DFT.[5] It also appears that a more posterior position of the left ventricular lead offers more advantage over an anterior position.[6]

> **Improvement in lead technology would likely include refinement in the design of current lead system as well as the development of new system using alternate cardiac positions**

Another alternative lead system is the combination of atrial and ventricular leads into a single lead. Several manufacturers have started to use this technology and the results of the clinical investigation will be available soon. Such a down-sizing may be greatly appreciated especially when multiple leads system will become a common approach in the future.

Improvement in ICD Operation

The software component of ICD has gained significant progress since the release of first prototype units almost two decades ago. The simple "shock box" has become a device with multiple choices for tachyarrhythmia therapy, complex detection schemes, and a "state-of-the-art" bradycardia pacemaker component. Naturally, the progress first involved refinement in the therapeutic scheme, followed by the addition of bradycardia therapy support and, subsequently, enhancement features in arrhythmia discrimination capability.

Improvement in Defibrillation

The therapeutic operational component of the device has been considered satisfactory since the inception of the concept of the implantable unit. The concern with insufficient safety margin of safety has been largely addressed by the advent of the more effective form of defibrillation using biphasic waveform. Defibrillation with ICD units using the biphasic waveform has been successful at energy levels that are much lower than the device's maximum output. It is uncommon to encounter a situation with a DFT greater than 20 joules. In most cases, when measured meticulously, the DFT is found to be between 5 and 15 joules. With most units capable of delivering 30 or 35 joules, the margin of safety is usually quite broad. The degree of confidence with being able to provide an excellent margin of safety is reflected in the abandonment of utilizing the external cardioverter-defibrillator (ECD) apparatus at implantation. Indeed, in our experience, we have never encountered a scenario where the ICD was not capable of terminating VF. Of the over 300 ICD units with biphasic waveform implanted between February 1995 through February 2000 in our institution, there was only five cases where the DFT was greater than 25 joules.

Among the various possibilities in the refinement in defibrillation delivery is in modifications of the defibrillation waveform. Variations to the reversal of waveform, such as triphasic waveform, were not shown to be advantageous.[7-9]

Other modification, such as the tilt, duration, and peak voltage of the first and/or second phase of the biphasic waveform appears to have some merit.[10,11] From relatively recent data showing that a lower tilt further improves defibrillation efficiency[10], some ICD units are now utilizing 50% instead of 65% while others offer the choice of either. There appears to be an interaction between the size of the capacitor, waveform, and tilt. The relative influence of each of these factors will need further studies to determine the most advantageous combination.

Other improvement currently in progress involves alteration in defibrillation lead and coil designs and modification in defibrillation pattern, such as using alternate anatomical position as discussed above. With these refinements, it would no longer be necessary to have the maximum output of the generator to be 30 or 35 joules. If a 20-joule device would be sufficient, the size of future pulse generator would be significantly smaller yet.

> Improvement in hardware technology would likely result in improvement in defibrillation efficacy, which in turn would result in improved efficiency and further reduction in pulse generator size

Refinement in Therapy for Ventricular Tachycardia

There has not been any significant progress in specific therapy for VT beyond antitachycardia pacing and low-energy cardioversion. The lack of progress in ATP therapy paralleled the absence of new insight into the understanding of the mechanism and behavior of the arrhythmia. Even if we accept the assumption that the mechanism is reentry (and there has been convincing experimental and clinical data to support that assumption), VT would behave significantly different from other simpler clinical reentrant arrhythmias such as AVNRT or AVRT. The substrate for VT in ischemic cardiomyopathy is generally diffused and therefore the response to ATP is variable and unpredictable. Furthermore, the patient with VT typically has significantly compromised underlying left ventricular function, even worse than patients with VF or nonsustained VT. Thus, prolonged attempts at ATP would result into progressive hypotension and increased proclivity to degeneration into VF. Only a better understanding of VT response to pacing would help in further utilization of ATP.

The efficacy of low-energy cardioversion has also been unpredictable and its risk of arrhythmia acceleration is not insignificant. Furthermore, its benefit is not clear. Typically, the patient would not be able to distinguish the pain of a 1-joule shock from that of a 35-joule shock. Thus, there is not likely to be any development or modification of these features.

The observation on the onset of VT has lead to some development in the management of VT. There have been reports by various investigators that polymorphic VT is frequently preceded by a short-long-short interval pattern. Prevention of sudden changes in ventricular cycle length is expected to reduce the likelihood for such polymorphic VT. Such preventive scheme can be implemented using pre-existing features such as Rate Smoothing or Ventricular Rate Stabilization. Further data on this specific VT pattern would likely result in the incorporation of such a feature.

Preventive pacing therapy for VT may also be available via other methods. Subthreshold stimulation may be of benefit, and such feature may also be useful in the prevention of VF. Multi-site pacing has also been postulated to provide a beneficial effect by creating a more synchronized pattern of depolarization and therefore prevent reentry. Although this has been shown to be potentially beneficial for the prevention of atrial fibrillation[12], its role in ventricular tachyarrhythma is unknown. However, there has been no data to show such benefit. In fact, there is also a concern for increasing the likelihood for VF using biventricular pacing, as shown in animal study.

> **Improvement in VT therapy is likely to occur in the field of tachycardia prevention**

Improvement in Tachyarrhythmia Detection

The new detection algorithm has significantly improved the ability to distinguish between ventricular and supraventricular tachyarrhythmia. The incorporation of dual-chamber sensing provides the essential tools for such discrimination. Assessment of EGM width or morphology has also proved to be useful and has improved the specificity significantly. This method of discrimination may become a common feature among all ICD. It is available in Ventritex, which is recently refined[13] and Medtronic units and is probably feasible with utilizing the shock electrode in CPI devices.[14]

However, all of those detection enhancement features utilize only electrical data. The significance of an arrhythmia also depends on its effect on hemodynamic status. Thus, even a supraventricular tachyarrhythmia may be potentially serious while a sustained ventricular tachycardia may be well tolerated. The status of hemodynamic stability and cerebral perfusion should also be taken into consideration.[15] Such information would be very useful in a therapeutic decision algorithm. Future improvement would therefore, likely incorporate parameters that would reflect the hemodynamic status of the patient if a central arterial pressure itself can not be continuously monitored. Of these, changes in the right atrial pressure and mixed venous oxygen concentration have been shown to reflect changes in central arterial pressure [16-19]. Alternatively, measurement of central arterial pressure may be able to be performed indirectly.

Further improvement in tachyarrhythmia detection may involve incorporation of other clinical variables that would directly or indirectly reflect the hemodynamic status during the arrhythmia

---

In addition to improvements in the method of tachyarrhythmia assessment, future devices will likely incorporate such a feedback automatically, thus providing a "closed loop" system. Such a system would greatly enhance the operation of an ICD in terms of providing comfort while preserving safety to the patient. However, the operation of such feedback system would need to be carefully designed and closely monitored.

The Incorporation of Therapy for Atrial Tachyarrhythmias

The Early Progress in Atrial Defibrillation Therapy

Automatic defibrillation for atrial fibrillation has been a major topic in the field of arrhythmia for several years. Although initially it received considerable attention, its role has been questioned. The reluctance in using this form of therapy stems from the combination of several factors. It was argued that patients would not likely desire or need a rapid treatment for atrial fibrillation with an internal shock because in most cases, the condition was considered as not deserving urgent intervention the patient, being minimally symptomatic, would not want to receive a painful shock. This reluctance was further substantiated by data that the "atrial DFT" was frequently in the "painful range" of 5 to 10 joules. For such reason, the clinical trial using the Metrix unit (InContol, Redmond, WA) included only patients with low atrial DFT of less than 4 joules.[20] Furthermore, it was feared that defibrillation of atrial fibrillation would risk the induction of ventricular tachyarrhythmia and therefore, a stand-alone atrial defibrillator was considered unsafe. It was estimated that only a small fraction of patients with AF would be good candidate for such therapy.[21]

The feasibility and practicality of the stand-alone device (an "atrioverter") was evaluated using the Metrix unit. This system utilizes two atrial defibrillation leads, positioned in the right atrium and coronary sinus, and a ventricular lead for shock synchronization. The patients selected were those with no significant underlying heart disease and having frequent AF episodes. The requirement of very low defibrillation threshold (mean of 1.5 J for model 3000 and 2.7 J for model 3200) excluded almost half of the patients enrolled. During the follow up period, 670 shocks were delivered for spontaneous AF in 51 patients with 41 patients experiencing at least one episode. The detection was 100% specific and 92% sensitive and the success rate was 96%. However, there were early recurrences noted in 27%of episodes and 51% of patients. Most importantly, there was no ventricular pro-arrhythmic outcome from the shocks.

The Dual-Chamber Atrioventricular Defibrillator

Electrical therapy for atrial tachyarrhythmia as part of an ICD, however, is perceived quite differently. The availability of such therapies within a (ventricular) ICD is now considered as a useful feature. Such a "renewed" interest may be the result of various developments in the field of arrhythmia. First of all, it is becoming increasingly recognized that atrial fibrillation may carry significant morbidity even if the event, by itself, may not cause significant symptom. The concern for thromboembolic complications and cardiovascular compromise that are related to atrial fibrillation has resulted in greater effort at preventing the progression of paroxysmal AF to persistent or chronic AF. As it is recognized that catheter ablative therapy is still of limited value in the permanent management of this arrhythmia, the interest in atrial defibrillation has re-emerged. Finally, the dual-defibrillation unit is probably more appropriate overall because the patient with underlying heart disease would likely have both types of tachyarrhythmia. Without the back up of ventricular defibrillation, the application of an automatic atrial defibrillation unit would probably be limited. Even in the patient without a history of ventricular tachyarrhythmia, there would still be a concern for the potential risk of pro-arrhythmia or the development of spontaneous VT/VF. In fact, in a recent study of the subset of AF patients without a history of VT, there was a surprisingly high incidence of spontaneous VF that was appropriately treated by the device. Vice versa, the patient receiving an ICD for VT/VF is likely to have a history of AF or develop atrial tachyarrhythmia in the future.[22]

Clinical Results

Significant amount of data is now available with respect to the efficacy, safety, and utility of the combined atrioventricular defibrillator, the Medtronic Jewel AF (Model 7250).[23-29]   With respect to its therapy for atrial tachyarrhythmia, in addition to shock treatment, this device provides three options of ATP that includes the usual Burst and Ramp, as well as a high frequency 50-Hz Burst pacing. This 50-Hz burst pacing was shown to be effective for atrial tachycardia as well as atrial fibrillation, thus further limiting the use of cardioversion.

A variety of defibrillation lead systems were tested. The initial approach was to use a coronary sinus lead in addition to the RA and RV lead. However, subsequent studies showed that the standard dual-chamber ICD lead system would be sufficient. In one study where a double coil RV defibrillation lead was used in combination with an atrial lead, a mean DFT of 5.4 J was achieved. In another study using the triad of RA, RV and the pulse generator, a higher mean DFT of 9.6 J was achieved with RV+RA→Can$^{(-)}$ and 16 J with RV→RA+Can$^{(-)}$ configuration.[30]

Detection accuracy in 80 patients with AT and AF was evaluated and recently reported [31]. AF detection window was programmed between 100 ms and 280 ms while AT detection window was between 180 ms and 320 ms. In the overlap zone, discrimination between AF and AT was performed based on regularity of the intervals. Detection accuracy was 98% for the 132 episodes of AF and 88% for the 190 episodes of AT.

Its therapy efficacy has been investigated in various scenario, including ATP (which includes 50-Hz burst) and low-energy cardioversion [30-33] showing good efficacy of ATP and shock therapy. For atrial tachycardia, which is defined as atrial arrhythmia with regular intervals, ATP (including 50-Hz burst) was effective in 45% to 85%.[31-33] Of the three types of ATPs, 50-Hz-Burst and Ramp were equally effective at 64% and 77%, respectively while simple Burst was relatively ineffective, at 15%.[33] Of interest, for arrhythmia declared as AF (based on irregular intervals), 50-Hz-Burst ATP was claimed to be effective in 15% to 20%.[32,34] The availability of ATP with 50-Hz Burst is a practical option of painless therapy. Low-energy cardioversion as the subsequent therapy was effective in over 90% of cases for AT but much lower (in the order of 60%) for AF.

The availability of telemetry and data retrieval from the current devices that incorporate atrial therapy also assists in the management of atrial tachyarrhythmias. The stability of recording and detecting atrial tachyarrhythmia can differentiate between atrial tachycardia and atrial fibrillation and deliver specific type and timing of therapies.[31,35]

> Atrial therapy will be available in the next generation ICD and this additional feature may be useful in a significant fraction of ICD patients, especially if some atrial fibrillation may indeed respond to 50-Hz burst pacing therapy

Pacing Therapy for Heart Failure

Rationale for Pacing Therapy

Pacing therapy was considered as a potential treatment of heart failure because these patients developed progressive conduction abnormalities, which were noted to have independent mortality prognostic values.[36-40] In the retrospective study by Wilensky et al[36], over 80% of the patients developed conduction abnormality. The PR interval would increase progressively, and in addition to the left ventricular ejection fraction, the development of 1st and 2nd degree AV block was noted to be an independent predictor of cardiovascular mortality.[37] Similarly, QRS widening was noted in a significant portion of patients with some reaching over 200 ms in duration before death [36].

The deleterious effects of conduction abnormalities may be due to various factors. Echocardiographic studies have shown the various abnormalities that are produced by atrioventricular delay and delayed left ventricular depolarization.[41,42] Thus, for instance, prolonged AV conduction would result in reduction in left atrial contribution to left ventricular filling and QRS widening would cause prolongation of LV isovolumetric contraction and relaxation time, impairing pumping action. The conduction abnormalities were also noted to cause mitral regurgitation.

Clinical Results

Thus, the role of pacing therapy for heart failure was investigated several years ago. Various parameters were assessed, such as shorter AV delay and, more recently, left ventricular pacing.[43-48] Clinical evaluation of feasibility, safety, and efficacy of biventricular pacing was then carried on independently by several investigators in Europe. Cazeau et al[43,45] studied the effects of biventricular pacing in 18 patients with advanced cardiomyopathy in NYHA functional class III or IV, with a mean QRS duration of 170 ms and PR interval of 220 ms. Significant improvement in cardiac output (from 2.0 L/min/m^2 to 2.7 L/min/m^2) and reduction in pulmonary capillary wedge pressure were noted, along with shortening of QRS duration from a baseline mean of 170 ms to 154 ms. In an earlier study conducted by Blanc et al[49], LV pacing produced similar hemodynamic benefits as biventricular pacing, while RV pacing alone did not. Similarly, a study utilizing echocardiographic parameters by Kass et al[50] also showed the superiority of LV pacing over RV and even biventricular. Of note, in this study by Kass et al, the AV delay parameter did not influence the outcome.

The preliminary results of the InSync and MIRACLE (Medtronic) study involving pacing therapy alone, which included several European and Canadian centers was published in 1998. The patients (43 in NYHA class III and 25 in class IV) were evaluated for changes in NYHA class, quality-of-life, six-minute walk tolerance, and LVEF. There was improvement in all categories although the increase in LVEF was not significant. There were 7 deaths from cardiovascular causes, including 4 sudden deaths. In their subsequent report[51], where 55 of 89 patients have had at least 6 months follow up, it was evident that there were sustained improvements in all categories, including LVEF (from a mean of 21% to 24%).

The incidence of sudden death has been a concern, given that these patients are also probably at increased risk for ventricular tachyarrhythmias. While the prevalence of sudden death can not yet be accurately determined at this time, it can be postulated that the "risk" for arrhythmia would be high in these patients cumulatively because of their improvement of heart failure status to a NYHA class with lower mortality from pump failure. Furthermore, it is also possible that biventricular pacing per se may be proarrhythmic. At the same time, ICD therapy alone in patients with significant heart failure may not offer significant benefit in overall mortality and quality-of-life. Hence, the combination therapy would appear to be a very logical approach for these patients.[52,53]   In a retrospective analysis of patients undergoing ICD implantation, Stellbrink et al[53] found that many of their patients would potentially benefit from pacing therapy, especially if those with NYHA class II were included. There are now several multi-center studies assessing the effect of combined pacing and ICD therapy in such patients (VENTAK-CHF, CONTAC-CD, InSync-ICD).   Of interest, there is an indication that in ICD patients, biventricular pacing may reduce the frequency of their arrhythmia[54] although others have shown the possibility of increased risk of arrhythmia.

Implementation of Biventricular Pacing

While there appears to be an agreement that patients with AV and LV conduction abnormalities would benefit from LV pacing, there is no general consensus on the most optimal method of pacing. The timing of AV delay remains a controversial issue. In one study[55], the investigators noted that a short AV delay would be potentially deleterious because it would result in simultaneous left atrial and ventricular depolarization, especially if there is inter-atrial conduction delay. In another study[56,57] however, the authors found that the shortest possible AV delay was most beneficial, as measured using echocardiographic study. Based on recent data, one finding that was associated with clinical improvement was the degree in QRS duration shortening with biventricular pacing compared to RV pacing only.[58] In such consideration, in the placement of the LV lead, the difference in paced QRS duration should be assessed. Such a site is also noted to have a marked delay in local depolarization during RV pacing (Figure 6-1).

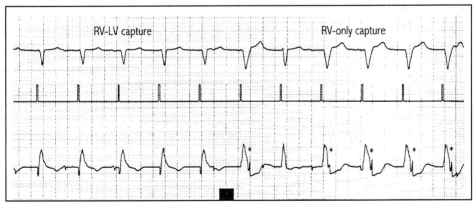

Figure 6-1. This figure shows the difference in QRS width during biventricular pacing (left side) and during RV pacing only, as pacing output is reduced (for threshold measurement). In this case, the QRS width during biventricular pacing (80 ms) was significantly narrower than during RV pacing (140 ms). It was also noted that there was a marked delay (160 ms) in depolarization of the LV pacing site after RV capture, as indicated by the asterisks (*).

At this stage, there is yet a uniform approach to the optimization of ventricular synchronization. While electrical parameters such as AV timing and QRS duration are shown to be useful parameters, it is not known whether there is a cause and effect association. It would be reasonable to also assess hemodynamic parameters but it would be difficult to determine which of the indirect parameters would be most useful. Further studies are obviously needed to determine the most predictive and accurate parameter.

There are also various methods of LV pacing. The choice is based primarily on the available tools and technique that is specific to the clinical protocol. Initial attempts at left ventricular pacing was performed via the thoracotomy approach, which offered the benefit of providing greater options of anatomical sites but was, naturally, associated with significant morbidity and mortality. The transvenous approach, using the coronary sinus and great cardiac venous placement of the ventricular lead has been associated with less serious complications but offers limited options with respect to anatomical positioning. Such implantation can be associated with significant technical difficulty. In their early experience, the success rate of implantation was only at 50 to 60%. Specially designed guide-wires and guiding catheters have improved the ease and success rate of implantation but the procedure still takes considerably longer than routine dual chamber pacemaker lead positioning. Furthermore, there is also a relatively higher rate of lead dislodgment.

In our experience, the advancement of the left ventricular lead via the coronary sinus approach would usually take the course of the direct tributary of the great cardiac vein, the anterior cardiac vein. This vein is normally located on the anterior portion of the left ventricle and may be at close proximity with the right ventricle. Thus, if the right ventricular catheter is located in the usual right ventricular apex position, there may be a relatively small distance between the two leads. In such configuration, there is frequently also a narrow interval between the timing of the right and left ventricular depolarizations and result in suboptimal re-synchronization. Indeed, in the cases where the LV lead was positioned in this close proximity, we noted only a modest narrowing of QRS duration with biventricular pacing compared to RV pacing.

It is also important to consider the means of pacing RV and LV simultaneously. In some systems, biventricular pacing is achieved by pacing both RV and LV using the same ventricular pacing output channel, while in others, RV and LV pacing can be programmed separately. While this may seem to be of little difference, it can pose some clinical decision issues. One issue involves the programming of pacing output. It should also be noted that there is usually a significant difference between the pacing capture thresholds of the two ventricular leads. The LV pacing capture threshold is commonly between one to two volts. Thus, if the two leads were to be connected to a single channel without differential programming, the pacing output must be programmed at a value that would assure capture of both ventricles. With the higher incidence of LV lead migration and dislodgment, the pacing output may need to be adjusted even to a higher value in some instances. Another issue is the possibility that LV pacing in some instances may be more beneficial than biventricular pacing.[59]

> Biventricular pacing therapy may reduce symptom and mortality from heart failure but as a result, whether directly or indirectly, may increase mortality from sudden death; hence, its incorporation into ICD would be a logical approach

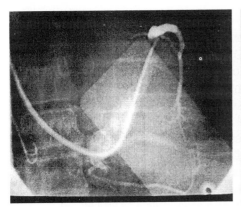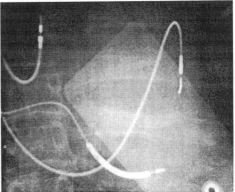

Figure 6-2. An anterior-posterior (AP) view of placement of a left ventricular pacing lead within the anterior cardiac vein (left panel). The placement was assisted by visualization of the venous tributaries using retrograde venography with antegrade occlusion. Note the presence of other large venous tributaries in the posterior region, which were visualized at a later phase because the inflated balloon typically "wedges" deep within the great cardiac vein. In this case, there was no posterolateral or lateral vein noted, which are believed to provide best locations for resynchonization. The right atrial and right ventricular (ICD) leads were placed afterwards.

It would seem logical to expect that biventricular pacing will become a feature of future ICD. The clinician must be prepared to deal with this issue in the implementation of ICD therapy. Screening is an essential component and at this point, without clear guidelines as the clinical parameters for accurate selection, this is not an easy step. Management of the patient, including device programming and problem solving may also be cumbersome. Furthermore, the additional lead itself may pose greater morbidity. It was noted that dual chamber ICD system has greater incidence of device and lead related complications than a single chamber unit[60] and naturally there are concerns with the use of multiple leads, especially if revision would become necessary.

Summary

The ICD has become the "complete" device for arrhythmia therapy and has reached a new platform in its stage of development. Many of its features have been refined, resulting in an improved performance in terms of withholding therapy for less serious arrhythmia while maintaining its efficacy in saving life. However, progress will likely continue and, furthermore, it will likely encompass greater scope of therapy. The next generations of ICD would likely become smaller but more complex in its operation. Therapy for atrial arrhythmia will likely become part of its scope. Other forms of pacing, such as those for arrhythmia prevention and treatment of heart failure will be soon incorporated. These additions may counterbalance the progress in miniaturization of the pulse generator and worse yet, sacrifice battery longevity. As such, the future generation of ICD may come in various packages and the clinician must choose the most appropriate one for the patient.

- With its current dual-chamber sensing, pacing and tachyarrhythmia therapy, the ICD has reached a new platform. However, it is likely to continue to improve. Its lead, battery, and capacitor technology will continue to be refined. Other modalities will also be available.
- Among the new modalities, atrial tachyarrhythmia therapy is a very useful one. Less painful therapy for atrial fibrillation with high-frequency burst pacing is effective in a surprisingly high percentage of patients. Early conversion of atrial tachyarrhythmia is also potentially beneficial in terms of increasing the likelihood of maintaining sinus rhythm as well as preventing atrial remodeling.
- New therapy for VT in the form of subthreshold inhibition may prove to be useful in preventing the occurrence of the tachycardia. Subthreshold pacing may even be beneficial in increasing contractility.
- Another new modality that is likely to be a common feature is bi-ventricular pacing for heart failure. So far clinical results are very favorable.
- Future devices are also likely to implement biosensors for feedback, which can be incorporated onto a closed loop system. Such closed loop system can integrate pacing, tachyarrhythmia, and heart failure therapies.

References

1. Swerdlow CD, Kass RM, O'Connor ME, *et al.* Effect of shock waveform on relationship between upper limit of vulnerability and defibrillation threshold. J Cardiovasc Electrophysiol, 1998;**9**(4):339-349.
2. Luria D, Rasmussen M, Hammill S, *et al.* Frequency and mode of detection of nonthoracotomy implantable defibrillator lead failure. PACE, 1999;**22**(4(II)):705.
3. Hauser R, Almquist A, and Kallinen L. Clinical reliability of implantable cardioverter defibrillator. PACE, 1999;**22**(4(II)):705.
4. Roberts P, Urban J, Euler D, *et al.* The midle cardiac vein - a novel pathway to reduce the defibrillation threshold. J Am Coll Cardiol, 1999;**33**(2):111A.
5. Meisel E, Butter C, Philippon F, *et al.* Human defibrillation using a transvenous left coronary vein lead and dual shock waveform: effect of left ventricular lead position. PACE, 1999;**22**(4(II)):699.
6. Yamanouchi Y, Efimov I, Hills D, *et al.* Biventricular defibrillation lead system significantly improved defibrillation efficacy. PACE, 1999;**22**(4(II)):699.
7. Dixon EG, Tang AS, Wolf PD, *et al.* Improved defibrillation thresholds with large contoured epicardial electrodes and biphasic waveforms. Circulation, 1987;**76**(5):1176-1184.
8. Sweeney RJ, Gill RM, Jones JL, *et al.* Defibrillation using a high-frequency series of monophasic rectangular pulses: observations and model predictions. J Cardiovasc Electrophysiol, 1996;**7**(2):134-143.
9. Walcott GP, Walker RG, Cates AW, *et al.* Choosing the optimal monophasic and biphasic waveforms for ventricular defibrillation. J Cardiovasc Electrophysiol, 1995;**6**(9):737-750.
10. Swerdlow CD, Kass RM, Davie S, *et al.* Short biphasic pulses from 90 microfarad capacitors lower defibrillation threshold. Pacing Clin Electrophysiol, 1996;**19**(7):1053-1060.
11. Tomassoni G, Newby K, Deshpande S, *et al.* Defibrillation efficacy of commercially available biphasic impulses in humans. Importance of negative-phase peak voltage. Circulation, 1997;**95**(7):1822-1826.
12. Ramdat Misier A, Beukema WP, and Oude Luttikhuis HA. Multisite or alternate site pacing for the prevention of atrial fibrillation. Am J Cardiol, 1999;**83**(5B):237D-240D.
13. Herwig S, Jung W, Wolpert C, *et al.* First result with a new morphology criterion dor discrimination of supraventricular and ventricular tachycardias. J Am Coll Cardiol, 2000:127A.
14. Chang A, Al-Ahmad A, Nunley S, *et al.* Can correlation waveform analysis of ICD shock electrograms be used to discriminate ventricular from supraventricular rhythms? J Am Coll Cardiol, 2000;**85**(2):128A.
15. Singer I and Edmonds H, Jr. Changes in cerebral perfusion during third-generation implantable cardioverter defibrillator testing. Am Heart J, 1994;**127**(4 Pt 2):1052-1057.
16. Cohen TJ. A theoretical right atrial pressure feedback heart rate control system to restore physiologic control to the rate-limited heart. Pacing Clin Electrophysiol, 1984;**7**(4):671-677.
17. Cohen TJ, Veltri EP, Lattuca JJ, *et al.* Hemodynamic responses to rapid pacing: a model for tachycardia differentiation. Pacing Clin Electrophysiol, 1988;**11**(11 Pt 1):1522-1528.
18. Cohen TJ and Liem LB. A hemodynamically responsive antitachycardia system. Development and basis for design in humans. Circulation, 1990;**82**(2):394-406.
19. Cohen TJ and Liem LB. Mixed venous oxygen saturation for differentiating stable from unstable tachycardias. Am Heart J, 1991;**122**(3 Pt 1):733-740.
20. Wellens HJ, Lau CP, Luderitz B, *et al.* Atrioverter: an implantable device for the treatment of atrial fibrillation. Circulation, 1998;**98**(16):1651-1656.
21. Seidl K, Drogenmuller A, Schwacke H, *et al.* How many patients are possible candidates for an implantable stand alone atrial cardioverter? Analysis of 694 patients with atrial fibrillation. J Am Coll Cardiol, 1999;**83**(2):146A.
22. Grimm W, Flores BF, and Marchlinski FE. Electrocardiographically documented unnecessary, spontaneous shocks in 241 patients with implantable cardioverter defibrillators. Pacing Clin Electrophysiol, 1992;**15**(11 Pt 1):1667-1673.
23. Carlson MD and Biblo LA. Atrial defibrillation. New frontiers. Cardiol Clin, 1996;**14**(4):607-622.
24. Cooklin M, Olsovsky M, Brockman R, *et al.* Comparison of atrial defibrillation thresholds with ventricular defibrillator lead configuration. Circulation, 1998;**98**(17):I-190.
25. Cooklin M, Shorofsky S, Olsovsky M, *et al.* Predictors of atrial defibrillation threshold in patients with single lead ICDs. Circulation, 1998;**98**(17):I-428.
26. Everett T, Moorman R, and Haines D. Prediction of successful intra-atrial defibrillation by analysis of atrial fibrillation waveform. Circulation, 1998;**98**(17):I-712.
27. Heisel A, Jung J, Fries R, *et al.* Atrial defibrillation: can modifications in current implantable cardioverter-defibrillators achieve this? Am J Cardiol, 1996;**78**(5A):119-127.

28.   Heisel A and Jung J. The atrial defibrillator: a stand-alone device or part of a combined dual-chamber system? Am J Cardiol, 1999;**83**(5B):218D-226D.

29.   Saksena S, Prakash A, Madan N, *et al.* New generations of implantable pacemaker defibrillators for ventricular and atrial tachyarrhythmias. Arch Mal Coeur Vaiss, 1996;**89 Spec No 1**:149-154.

30.   Chaudry G, Warman E, Casavant D, *et al.* Optimization of atrial defibrillation pathways without use of coronary sinus leads in patients receiving Medtronic 7250 dual chamber defibrillator (Jewel AF). J Am Coll Cardiol, 2000;**85**(2):104A.

31.   Swerdlow CD, Schsls W, Dijkman B, *et al.* Detection of Atrial Fibrillation and Flutter by a Dual-Chamber Implantable Cardioverter-Defibrillator. Circulation, 2000;**101**(8):878-885.

32.   Ricci R, Pandozi C, Altamura G, *et al.* Efficacy of anti-tachy-pacing (ATP) therapies and low energy cardioversion in terminating spontaneous atrial tachyarrhythmias in patients with dual implantable defibrillator. J Am Coll Cardiol, 2000;**85**(2):104A.

33.   Rameken M, Schwacke H, Siemon G, *et al.* Atrial tachyarrhythmias in patients with a dual-chamber cardioveter-defibrillator: efficacy of atrial therapies. J am Coll Cardiol, 2000;**85**(2):10A.

34.   Gold M, Daubert J, Peters R, *et al.* A clinical trial of a combined atrial and ventricular defibrillator in patients without ventricular arrhythmia. J Am Coll Cardiol, 2000;**85**(2):115A.

35.   Wolpert C, Jung W, Tenzer D, *et al.* Duration and circadian variation of paroxysmal atrial tachyarrhythmias in patients with dual chamber implantable defibrillator: implications for programming of atrial therapies. J Am Coll Cardiol, 1999;**83**(2):159A.

36.   Wilensky RL, Yudelman P, Cohen AI, *et al.* Serial electrocardiographic changes in idiopathic dilated cardiomyopathy confirmed at necropsy. Am J Cardiol, 1988;**62**(4):276-283.

37.   Schoeller R, Andresen D, Buttner P, *et al.* First- or second-degree atrioventricular block as a risk factor in idiopathic dilated cardiomyopathy. Am J Cardiol, 1993;**71**(8):720-726.

38.   Likoff MJ, Chandler SL, and Kay HR. Clinical determinants of mortality in chronic congestive heart failure secondary to idiopathic dilated or to ischemic cardiomyopathy. Am J Cardiol, 1987;**59**(6):634-638.

39.   Cowburn PJ, Cleland JG, Coats AJ, *et al.* Risk stratification in chronic heart failure. Eur Heart J, 1998;**19**(5):696-710.

40.   Silverman ME, Pressel MD, Brackett JC, *et al.* Prognostic value of the signal-averaged electrocardiogram and a prolonged QRS in ischemic and nonischemic cardiomyopathy. Am J Cardiol, 1995;**75**(7):460-464.

41.   Nishimura RA, Hayes DL, Holmes DR, Jr., *et al.* Mechanism of hemodynamic improvement by dual-chamber pacing for severe left ventricular dysfunction: an acute Doppler and catheterization hemodynamic study. J Am Coll Cardiol, 1995;**25**(2):281-288.

42.   Xiao HB, Brecker SJ, and Gibson DG. Effects of abnormal activation on the time course of the left ventricular pressure pulse in dilated cardiomyopathy. Br Heart J, 1992;**68**(4):403-407.

43.   Cazeau S, Ritter P, Lazarus A, *et al.* Multisite pacing for end-stage heart failure: early experience. Pacing Clin Electrophysiol, 1996;**19**(11 Pt 2):1748-1757.

44.   Gras D, Mabo P, Tang T, *et al.* Multisite pacing as a supplemental treatment of congestive heart failure: preliminary results of the Medtronic Inc. InSync Study. Pacing Clin Electrophysiol, 1998;**21**(11 Pt 2):2249-2255.

45.   Leclercq C, Cazeau S, Le Breton H, *et al.* Acute hemodynamic effects of biventricular DDD pacing in patients with end-stage heart failure. J Am Coll Cardiol, 1998;**32**(7):1825-1831.

46.   Auricchio A, Stellbrink C, Sack S, *et al.* The Pacing Therapies for Congestive Heart Failure (PATH-CHF) study: rationale, design, and endpoints of a prospective randomized multicenter study. Am J Cardiol, 1999;**83**(5B):130D-135D.

47.   Ansalone G, Trambaiolo P, Giorda GP, *et al.* Multisite stimulation in refractory heart failure. G Ital Cardiol, 1999;**29**(4):451-459.

48.   Saxon LA, Boehmer JP, Hummel J, *et al.* Biventricular pacing in patients with congestive heart failure: two prospective randomized trials. The VIGOR CHF and VENTAK CHF Investigators. Am J Cardiol, 1999;**83**(5B):120D-123D.

49.   Blanc JJ, Etienne Y, Gilard M, *et al.* Evaluation of different ventricular pacing sites in patients with severe heart failure: results of an acute hemodynamic study. Circulation, 1997;**96**(10):3273-3277.

50.   Kass DA, Chen CH, Curry C, *et al.* Improved left ventricular mechanics from acute VDD pacing in patients with dilated cardiomyopathy and ventricular conduction delay. Circulation, 1999;**99**(12):1567-1573.

51.   Leclercq C, Alonso C, Pavin D, *et al.* Single-center experience withtransvenous biventricular pacing to treat advance heart failure:long-term clinical results. J Am Coll Cardiol, 2000;**85**(2):116A.

52.   Le Franc P, Klug D, Lacroix D, *et al.* Triple chamber pacemaker for end-stage heart failure in a patient with a previously implanted automatic defibrillator. Pacing Clin Electrophysiol, 1998;**21**(8):1672-1675.

53.   Stellbrink C, Auricchio A, Diem B, *et al.* Potential benefit of biventricular pacing in patients with congestive heart failure and ventricular tachyarrhythmia. Am J Cardiol, 1999;**83**(5B):143D-150D.

54.   Higgins S, Yong P, Scheck D, *et al.* Biventricular pacing may diminish ICD shocks. PACE, 1999;**22**(4(II)):848.

55.   Saxon L, Hourigan L, Guerra P, *et al.* Influence of programmed AV delay on left ventricularperformance in biventricular pacing systems for treatment of heart failure. J Am Coll Cardiol, 2000;**85**(2):116A.

56.   Breithardt O, Stellbrink C, Franke A, *et al.* Acute effect of multisite pacing with different atrioventricular delays on the non-invasive doppler-derived myocardial performance index (MPI). J Am Coll Cardiol, 2000;**85**(2):117A.

57.   Breithardt O, Stellbrink C, Franke A, *et al.* Non-invasive determination of optimal pacing site by doppler echocardiography in comparisonto invasive hemodynamic testing: results ofthe PATH-CHF study. J Am Coll Cardiol, 2000;**85**(2):117A.

58.   Gras D, Mabo P, Bucknall C, *et al.* Responders and nonresponders to cardiac resynchronization therapy: results from the InSync trial. J Am Coll Cardiol, 2000;**85**(2):230A.

59.   Bradley K, Florio J, Pianca A, *et al.* Hemodynamic comparison of left ventricular and biventricular pacing. PACE, 1999;**22**(4(II)):901.

60.   Takahashi T, Cannom D, Abdullah E, *et al.* Dual-chamber implantable cardioverter defibrillator vs single-chamber implantable cardioverter defibrillator: high incidence of device and lead related complications in dual-chamber implantable cardioverter defibrillator. J Am Coll Cardiol, 2000;**85**(2):127A.

Index

A

W